the blink of an eye

a memoir of dying—and learning how to live again

Rikke Schmidt Kjærgaard

Foreword by Bill Bryson

THE EXPERIMENT

NEW YORK

Originally published in Great Britain as *The Blink of an Eye: How I Died and Started Living* by Hodder & Stoughton, a Hachette UK company, in 2018.
First published in North America by The Experiment, LLC, in 2019.

The Experiment, LLC, 220 East 23rd Street, Suite 600, New York, NY 10010-4658
theexperimentpublishing.com

This book contains the opinions and ideas of its author. It is intended to provide helpful and informative material on the subjects addressed in the book. It is sold with the understanding that the author and publisher are not engaged in rendering medical, health, or any other kind of personal professional services in the book. The author and publisher specifically disclaim all responsibility for any liability, loss, or risk—personal or otherwise—that is incurred as a consequence, directly or indirectly, of the use and application of any of the contents of this book.

Many of the designations used by manufacturers and sellers to distinguish their products are claimed as trademarks. Where those designations appear in this book and The Experiment was aware of a trademark claim, the designations have been capitalized.

The Experiment's books are available at special discounts when purchased in bulk for premiums and sales promotions as well as for fund-raising or educational use. For details, contact us at info@theexperimentpublishing.com.

Library of Congress Cataloging-in-Publication Data

Names: Kjaergaard, Rikke Schmidt, author.
Title: The blink of an eye : a memoir of dying--and learning how to live
   again / Rikke Schmidt Kjaergaard.
Description: New York, NY : The Experiment, LLC, 2019. | Previous title: The
   blink of an eye: how I died and started living. 2018.
Identifiers: LCCN 2019004727 (print) | LCCN 2019008568 (ebook) | ISBN
   9781615195725 (ebook) | ISBN 9781615195718 (pbk.)
Subjects: LCSH: Kjaergaard, Rikke Schmidt,--Health. | Kjaergaard, Rikke
   Schmidt,--Family. | Streptococcus
   pneumoniae--Patients--Rehabilitation--Biography. | Streptococcus
   pneumoniae--Patients--Family relationships--Biography. | Physician and
   patient.
Classification: LCC QR82.S78 (ebook) | LCC QR82.S78 K53 2019 (print) | DDC
   579.3/55--dc23
LC record available at https://lccn.loc.gov/2019004727

ISBN 978-1-61519-571-8
Ebook ISBN 978-1-61519-572-5

Cover design by Beth Bugler | Text design by Sarah Schneider | Cover and author photograph by Katrine Philp

Manufactured in the United States of America

First printing May 2019
10 9 8 7 6 5 4 3 2 1

To Daniel, Victoria and Johan,
who showed remarkable courage.
To Peter, who never left my side.

With love and admiration.

Contents

Foreword

BY BILL BRYSON

In the winter of 2016, as part of a project I was involved in, I spent some time at the Natural History Museum of Denmark in Copenhagen. One evening, after a long day at the museum, I went for dinner with my host, a genial English-born geneticist named Tom Gilbert. At the last moment we were joined by his boss, the museum's director, Peter C. Kjærgaard.

I had only met Peter that day, but I liked him immediately, as I imagine most people do. He is clearly superintelligent, but also charming and kindly, with a distinctly approachable manner. If you were lost in a strange city, he is the person you would ask for directions.

Early in the dinner, Peter's phone rang, and he asked if we minded very much if he took the call. His wife had been ill, he explained, and he wanted to be sure she was all right.

We assured him, of course, that he should speak to her. Their conversation was brief and murmured, as you would expect in a restaurant, but the news was evidently good. Peter looked pleased, and indeed relieved, as he returned the phone to his pocket and told us all was well.

Tom or I said something to the effect that we hoped it was nothing too serious.

"Well, actually, she has been really quite unwell," Peter responded rather suddenly. He hesitated, as if unsure whether to go on, then proceeded to tell us the most spellbinding and harrowing story I believe I have ever heard. It is the story you are about to read.

I don't wish to give away a single detail of what follows. It is Rikke Schmidt Kjærgaard's story to tell, and no one could tell it better or more feelingly. I will just say that I met Rikke soon afterward and liked her immediately, too. She has much the same qualities as Peter—she is gracious and urbane, kindly, a good listener, very learned, deeply and obviously devoted to family. I can say at once with confidence that you would like her very much yourself.

She has given us a most exceptional book, and exceptional in many ways. At its most immediate level, it is a calm, measured, impeccably lucid account of a truly horrifying experience told from the all-too-rare perspective of the sufferer. Rikke is a scientist by background, and she recounts the details of her ordeal with a kind of forensic precision that makes the horror of the experience all the more vivid and chilling. No one should have to go through what she did, but you could hardly choose a more skilled and insightful victim.

But this is much more—much, much more—than a clinical record of a terrible experience. It is above all a highly personal, deeply affecting account of what it is to be yanked from a happy, well-ordered life and thrust into a sudden, unimaginable, terrifying darkness. Rikke has done the impossible of putting into words an experience that would seem to be beyond expressing.

And she has done it with the most abundant generosity. This is at its heart a book about familial bonds. Nothing says more for Rikke's character, as both writer and person, than that you come away profoundly touched not only by the wearisome awfulness of her ordeal, but by the emotional and physical fortitude of Peter and her children. This was, from beginning to end, a shared horror.

Perhaps the most extraordinary thing about this book is that it exists at all. What happened to Rikke is not as rare as we might think or hope. No one knows how many people in the world exist in comas or are otherwise "minimally conscious," as the medical jargon has it. Almost nowhere are records systematically kept. But according to the journal *Nature Neuroscience,* the number globally is in the hundreds of thousands. Few of those poor people will ever be able to resume normal lives.

Rikke Schmidt Kjærgaard is a brave and lovely exception. As *The Blink of an Eye* proves, we are lucky, in every sense of the word, to have her.

BILL BRYSON's bestselling books include *A Walk in the Woods, I'm a Stranger Here Myself, In a Sunburned Country,* and *A Short History of Nearly Everything.*

ONE

Dying

My death could not have been predicted. It came suddenly. I was my usual self the day before. We'd had houseguests for New Year's Eve and spent the evening chatting, singing, playing music, and eating great food. We stood to toast 2013 circled around the TV, sharing in the drama of the Bell Tower of Copenhagen City Hall's countdown to midnight. I loved that magic beat between the last second of the old year and the first one of the new: the micropause between the past and future, the promise and the expectations. Later, I tumbled into bed, full of happiness and celebration.

The following morning we were still in a festive mood. It was a beautiful day. Cool, clear winter with just enough snow to cover the ground, and frozen puddles waiting to crack from the force of a child's playful jump. We went for a walk along the river near our house. We lived in a large Danish town; a nice, somewhat sleepy place. We'd bought the house several years earlier, shortly before our youngest son, Daniel, was born. We had moved from a larger university city further south, because we wanted more space and a garden for our three children.

Over the years we had worked on it, knocking down walls and building new ones, laying new floorboards and painting everything in light colors. This was the first place we had owned and we had made it ours. When our jobs took us abroad for several years, we kept the house, coming back for the summer holidays, which made Daniel think that Denmark was a land of perpetual summers. I loved our house. When storms raged, if we had bad news to cope with or stressful days, our home was where we retreated. It was our haven. A safe place where nothing bad could happen.

The river we were strolling along ran all the way to the sea. The kids raced along the track: Johan, just eighteen and home on visit from his studies in Hong Kong, and Victoria, four years younger, two teenagers following their younger brother's lead, forgetting how busy they were growing up. My husband, Peter, was deep in conversation with an old friend and colleague from England, who had stayed with us overnight. Watching from a distance, I saw him waving his arms in the air, a gesture so familiar to me it almost felt like my own. I had seen this many times before, when he was making a point or putting a funny spin on a serious topic.

Peter is a charmer, eloquent and charismatic. From the very first time I met him, I admired his immediate way of engaging with people and making them feel special. We had met at a university Christmas party where we'd been paired up for a science quiz, completely by chance. Pure luck. We'd won. "We make a great team, you and I, don't you think?" he'd said.

Walking along the banks of the river I felt chilly, cold through to my bones. My limbs felt leaden and heavy. Nobody noticed I was lagging behind. I tried to catch up but couldn't. I wanted to call Peter, but I felt as if I had run out of air. I dismissed it. Everybody feels a bit tired on New Year's Day. Moments later, Daniel, our eight-year-old happy, carefree boy, came running to hide behind me so the others wouldn't catch him. As Victoria tagged her father and they all ran circles around me, laughing, I just stood there, smiling at their playfulness.

Back home, I was still feeling cold. As everyone dispersed around the house, I went straight in to run myself a bath and lay in the hot water, wondering why I couldn't get warm. I wanted to make sure my body temperature stabilized. When I was twenty, I had been diagnosed with SLE—*systemic lupus erythematosus*—a chronic auto-immune disease where the cells of the immune system mistakenly attack healthy tissue. Having SLE means you are more prone to being ill, and even though I wasn't receiving medical treatment for it any more, having lived with the risks and necessary provisions to stay healthy for so many years, the fear of having relapses and severe recurrences still frightened me. If my temperature rose noticeably and for longer periods of time, I had to call a doctor.

Besides occasional joint pain and tiredness, I was not usually bothered by the illness. It really wasn't a condition that interfered with my life. Sore fingers or wrists, or a mild butterfly rash on my cheeks and the bridge of my nose, were signs of exhaustion and lack of rest and indicated activity in the illness. I knew I had to take these seriously and would give myself a break when they surfaced. When I'd first been diagnosed, I quickly decided that I would not let myself be sick, that I would still be able to live my life to the fullest.

Now though, this sudden inability to get warm made me mildly nervous. As I got out of the bath, I was shivering. My muscles were working hard, rapidly contracting and relaxing, and I could not seem to generate any heat in my body. I lay on the bed and called Peter.

"Could you get me a couple of blankets, please?" I asked him.

"Are you feeling OK?"

I decided I didn't have to answer him.

Piling blankets over me, Peter looked worried. That special look he gets when something is not right.

"I'm still freezing." My teeth were chattering and my limbs were shaking.

Peter called for Johan to bring a couple of duvets, and together they laid them on top of me. I didn't have the heart to tell them that I still felt as if I was lying in a bed of ice.

Night comes early in Scandinavian winter. At four in the afternoon, the bedroom lights were on and the brightness felt like icicles piercing my eyes. I asked Peter to turn off the lights and managed to tell him I would call him if I needed anything.

"OK. I'll let you get some rest then." But he left the door open on his way out.

My temperature continued to drop. As each hour went by, it felt like days. The house was quiet, subdued, as if everything had been turned down to a lower volume for me. Maybe they were also tired after the New Year celebrations? Daniel was probably playing with his Legos, Victoria reading, Johan and Peter preparing supper. I decided it must be the same thing for me, and that I had caught a common cold. Nothing serious.

But then the fever hit. I lay there freezing cold, shivering one minute and shaking with fever the next, my temperature shooting up and down. My thoughts became muddled and loud. Was it a school day tomorrow? What did the children need? I wanted to get up and pack their school bags.

I was dimly aware of the children coming to say good-night and then Peter being in bed. For a brief moment, I was able to register that he was talking, but then felt a desperate need to empty my bowels and I lost all sense of what he was saying. Victoria came out of her room and stood in the hallway watching her father carry me to the bathroom, Johan helping to support me. The sense that something was seriously wrong hung in the air. I wanted to tell them everything was going to be all right, but succumbed to body cramps. Peter closed the door gently, providing me with privacy I was too sick to care about.

My body exploded with vomit and diarrhea. I was delirious with fever and the few times I surfaced, I tried to tell Peter that if I could be left alone for a while, I would be fine, and if he would stop making all that noise, I would feel better. But Peter was silent. The noise was my retching, the deep growling of a body in pain.

For a moment, I suddenly felt better. "No need for a doctor," I said. "Let me rest. Get some sleep yourself. I'll call you if I need you." But before he could answer, another explosion sent me even further down than before.

"Rikke, I'm calling the doctor," he said, firmly.

I didn't really pay any attention to Peter's meticulous explanations on the phone, but apparently they worked. The GP on night duty took the house call.

Waddling through the house, keeping his muddy shoes on, he shot me one tired glance.

"It's the flu," he said. "Everybody's got the flu. Sit up straight. You'll be fine."

Turning to Peter, he said, "I'll put in a prescription for Tamiflu. Make her take it and see your own GP in the morning." Then he left.

What do you *do* in such a situation? The doctor had told Peter it was the flu, and to go and get me some Tamiflu. Not being a medical doctor himself, how could he do otherwise? But Peter knew something was terribly wrong. He had told the doctor about my SLE. He could see that my body was collapsing, that I couldn't sit up as the doctor had commanded, that I couldn't eat or drink, that I was way past the point of being able to control the vomiting and diarrhea. But he could only go on the on-call doctor's medical opinion that it was nothing to worry about. He went off to pick up the prescription at the night chemist.

The Tamiflu made no difference. I could not even keep water down, let alone the pill itself. And as the endless night wore on, the fever and constant vomiting were taking their toll. Peter was exhausted from cleaning up after me, changing and washing sheets, carrying me back and forth to the bathroom in a seemingly endless march. I could sense the restlessness in the house, Johan and Victoria initially tiptoeing around to check what was going on, and then as I got worse and worse, lying worried and awake in their beds. Only Daniel had fallen into a restless sleep.

In the early morning, my vomit turned black. Dark and thick. I couldn't even move my head to reach the bucket. I tried to keep going by forcing myself to answer Peter's questions, but he couldn't make any sense of what I was saying. Scared out of his wits, he called our surgery the moment it opened, to urge our GP to come immediately. Sensing the panic in Peter's voice, the receptionist promised to get hold of our doctor as quickly as possible.

Later, we learned that our GP hesitated when that call came. Out with his family and some friends, he was enjoying a last morning of the New Year break. He thought about not picking up but, ever diligent, he took the call.

With a biological storm hammering its way through my last defenses, that was my lucky break.

"Rikke! Can you hear what I'm saying?" I could hear someone breathing heavily, words as if they were coming from far away. The voice got louder. "Peter. This is not good. Try to straighten her arm."

My body seized up. The GP injected a dose of penicillin into my arm while Peter tried to hold it still. A syringe fell onto the ceramic tiles in the bedroom.

Within minutes two ambulances arrived. Paramedics ran through the house, shouting, pushing furniture aside, here to save a life.

I didn't sense the paramedics moving me. I was leaving. Strapped to a stretcher, my heart slowed down. And then, it stopped.

I was clinically dead.

There was nothing. No light at the end of the tunnel, no angels, no harps. No Heaven's Gate and no Hell. Nothing. Being dead means exactly that. You are gone. It's as simple and frightening as that.

My heart may have stopped, but the paramedics were not going to give up that easily. While in the ambulance, they worked on me, urging me to stay with them. However, as they pumped my heart into beating, the rest of my organs began to surrender. You can only push nature so far. My body was beginning to come to the end of its life.

Turning to Peter, our GP said, "You can't drive. You're in shock. I'll take you. Leave the children with your mother and she can bring them in her car."

Peter's mother had arrived shortly before the ambulances to help out. In a kind of dreamlike trance, Peter took the front seat in our GP's car.

"I'm sorry, I can't tell you exactly what's going to happen," said our GP. "It's a matter of minutes. It might still be possible to save her, and that we got to her just in time."

As I was being transferred from the ambulance to Intensive Care, doctors were ready with a defibrillator to send tiny electrical shocks into my heart in an attempt to restore its rhythm. I was put on a ventilator to get air into my lungs, and a dialysis machine to clean my blood. There was really nothing left now that I could do myself. I was pricked and pierced, but little did it matter. Not even my bodily reflexes worked. I had entered a passive, comatose state of peace. A deep state of unconsciousness, away from the turmoil.

From somewhere far away, the very bottom of the sea maybe, I could hear a nurse call my name: "Rikke, Rikke. Your children are here."

"Hi, Mummy!" came a barely audible, tiny voice.

And then, miraculously, before my brain shut down completely, it reacted by allowing one last salty, watery signal as my children touched me, three different sized hands stroking my arm. What remained of my conscious mind said goodbye with a solitary tear to the tiny group of people I loved the most in the world.

And then I sank into the darkness.

Victoria's small voice filled the room as she reached for her father's hand. "What will happen to Mum?"

"I don't know, sweetheart. I don't know," he said. Victoria flinched. Her father always had answers.

TWO

Surviving

It was a nurse in Intensive Care who told Peter, "Write down a few notes about what happens every day. If you write things down, it will help you remember." What she meant, but what she couldn't quite bring herself to say, was: Write everything down so that you will have something to remember your wife by when she is gone.

Peter is a university professor and an expert in human history, the very deep history that takes us back millions of years to our ape ancestry. Documenting is second nature to him, and he is never without a pen and notepad. An acute observer of everyday life, he lets no detail escape him, and so this advice resonated. He began to chart everything, meticulously documenting all the things that happened and the emotional responses of the children, of our extended family, and his own deepest, most private thoughts. And as the days darkened, Peter knew that I would want to know everything—and if not me, then the children, who would want to know in time, if the very worst happened.

Writing kept him sane.

His notes were what enabled me to piece this time together. Like much of this story of the days before I got sick and the weeks that followed, I've had to fit it all together, like writing a biography of another person. Doctor's notes. Medical charts. Endless readings of my bodily functions. Doses of drugs. Photographs. X-rays. Scans. All the records I could get my hands on. Conversations with staff. Physicians. Nurses. Therapists. Family. Friends.

A nurse had taken Peter aside and told him that "in situations like this," all close family members should be there. "What *is* a situation like this?" asked Peter. "Are those her parents?" replied the nurse, looking over at Peter's parents, who had arrived earlier and brought the children to the hospital. When Peter shook his head, she advised him to call my parents and "any other close family" right now. Seeing Peter's expression, she offered to make the call.

My parents divorced after I moved away from home to go to college. My younger sister now had her own family.

My father had a new one. My mother married again, too, but was now living alone. But they all still lived close to each other; I was the odd one out, living away from everyone else.

"You need to come immediately," the nurse told my mum. "You should be prepared to say goodbye." My mother broke down, completely unable to take in what the nurse was telling her. Nothing made sense. At least Peter had witnessed my collapse. To my mother and then my sister and father, there was nothing wrong. They had all talked to me the day before. What did the nurse mean they had to say goodbye?

Meanwhile, a decision was made to scan my brain. It was a risk. I might have already been too fragile, and simply moving me to the scanner could have had fatal consequences. But there was no way around it at this stage. The doctors needed to see how severe the damage was, to check if I was brain dead. In a body that was now a biological battlefield, with armies of blood clots pounding away at any remaining healthy part, this would be a highly probable scenario. If that was the case and I had already mentally departed, never to return, swift action was required to harvest whatever useful organs were still left in my body to save others. Following the scan, doctors thought there was still a chance I might make it, but not at the local hospital. Instead, I needed to be taken to the university hospital, a leading research facility thirty miles south. Before the doctors had a chance to discuss this with Peter, I was on my way.

To prevent whatever it was that had hit me from spreading and sending the others down the same perilous road, Peter and the children had to take a powerful antidote against the most aggressive of bacterial infections. For Peter, Johan, and Victoria, this made total sense; but for Daniel, in his confusion and shock, taking pills was not something he was able to do. In his eight-year-old mind, all he could see were enemies—illness, the hospital, doctors, nurses—who had so suddenly taken his mother away from him, and he believed instinctively that in order to save me and himself, he needed to fight them with everything he had.

Peter tried to comfort Daniel, but was getting increasingly desperate. He knew that I was probably dying, and at the same time he was fighting for this not to happen to any other member of the family. He knew he had to get Daniel to take that medicine.

Two doctors, two nurses, two hours. Pills, sugar-coated and yogurt-enhanced, broken and crushed. Persuasion, cajoling, bribing. Nothing seemed to work. But in the end, Daniel caved in and, because time now was of the essence, had a double dose injected straight into his veins. He was safe.

As I was being transferred from the local hospital to the university hospital, the health authorities were following protocol and had already started damage control. Immediate family had been taken care of. The next step was to track down our houseguests from New Year's Eve. They were already far away in the Netherlands and in Britain. To ensure their safety, they, too, needed shots.

While I was being settled into a bed in Intensive Care, isolated from all other patients, my father-in-law drove Peter, his mother, and the children to the university hospital, where they were joined by my parents and sister, who had by now driven the two and a half hours across the country. A doctor had come to tell them what she knew of my condition.

It was already dark outside. The night shift was in place. A workday like any other at Intensive Care.

My sister was the first to speak. "I just need to know one thing. Will she still be here tomorrow?"

"We can't tell," the doctor said.

Victoria froze. Fourteen—perceptive and sensitive—she made the connection between now and the next day when I might not be there. She kept her gaze fixed firmly on her father, hoping he could give her what the doctor did not. Her heart broke. Going to bed was all of a sudden dangerous, because waking up could bring the most terrifying news, and so, without saying a word, she made a decision not to sleep. Irrational as it was, in that moment, she believed her way of helping me to live was to fight her own need for sleep. And so began her own difficult internal battle.

My body was in septic shock and had started the process of killing itself. Multiple micro blood clots were exploding inside me like tiny fireworks, while small blood vessels started to leak everywhere. My body was bloated, already forty pounds heavier from the fluids being pumped into me; my hands, feet, and nose were turning black. My face and the rest of my body were purple, blue, and dark red, as a mosaic pattern grew from deep beneath my skin. I was in a deep coma.

My medication was controlled by what was literally called a space station, fitted with super-advanced devices constantly monitoring and administering high-precision, computer-controlled dosages. There was everything you know from the movies or your favorite medical drama series, only more of everything. All the lights, screens, tubes and wires feeding my carefully balanced intravenous medical cocktail, making sure I got just enough of everything and not too little. Even a small mistake could tip me over the edge.

I was being treated for an aggressive bacterial infection, but so far that was only the doctors' best bet. I could have had an aggressive virus, or even a rare parasite or a malignant fungus. I was still in quarantine, and so to be in the same room, but not contaminated by me, visitors and medical staff had to go through a complex routine, disinfecting hands, putting on disposable medical coveralls and facemasks.

Involuntary actors in a science fiction movie, my children were reluctant to set foot in my room. They were terrified. I was barely recognizable and I was barely alive. Johan was the first to muster the courage. Standing next to his father, wearing strange protective clothing so as not to be condemned to a terrible fate by his mother, my son watched. He knew that I was being kept artificially alive, against all hope and odds.

On the first night, Victoria made it to the doorway. She didn't want to come in. She peeked through the door to catch a glimpse of my bed. She hardly saw me. It was even more difficult for Daniel. He could scarcely manage to hear about how I was doing. He couldn't even bear to see the door of the room I was in. On the third day, after Peter had taken them to the maternity unit in which they were born, and they had been able to forget the real world for a moment, they gained the strength to come in and stand by my bed, talking, crying, watching.

While I was totally unaware of what was happening, it soon became clear to Peter that something was upsetting Daniel above and beyond the trauma of seeing me, and when he burst into uncontrollable tears, Peter took him outside. They walked into the quiet winter darkness, holding hands. There, his tiny body shaking, he told his father, "I'm scared of mobile phones."

Nobody had noticed his silent pain. After a while, as his father held him tight, he calmed down. And then it came out: In the face of such mystification and shock, all he could do was to watch what was going on. To watch me, to watch the doctors and nurses, to watch the machines, to watch his father, his sister and brother, his grandparents, his aunt. From his eight-year-old perspective, he was literally looking up and observing and all he could see were grief-stricken faces. Adults crying. Seeing how they crumbled in the hall outside my room. Seeing how they were trying but ultimately failing to control themselves, how they fell apart. Seeing how they stopped noticing him, because all they saw was me.

Barely audible, his voice was but a tiny whisper.

"Every time a phone rings, I'm afraid someone will tell me Mum has died."

Eight years old, he didn't own a phone, but everyone around him did and they were using them. Constantly. They were talking about me. He heard adults crying on the phone. He heard them telling others that I probably wouldn't survive. From the mobile phone conversations we all think go unheard, he picked up everything. People around me expected me to die. But no one told him this to his face, so he had to put the pieces together for himself. And he arrived at the inevitable conclusion. It was just a matter of when. The way the message would be delivered was already obvious. The sound of a mobile phone was the sound of the end.

At the university hospital, Peter was told not to be more than a few minutes away from me. I was never alone—there was a nurse with me twenty-four hours a day. The nights were often filled with insecurity and new medical examinations. Suddenly my blood pressure would rise or my temperature would drop. The saturation of my blood would fall, and my heart rate slow down. Nurses and doctors would rush in. In thirty seconds things could go from calm to nerve-wracking chaos. There would be new tests and waiting. Lots of waiting. Changing bags of blood and plasma, giving me a new run of saline, all of this, unnatural as it would have been only days before, became the new normal. Spending all of his waking hours by my side, in the same room with everything going on around me, Peter began to go with the routines.

The hospital had rooms for friends and relatives of severely or terminally ill patients. It was like a hotel—but then again, it was nothing like a hotel. Peter checked in. During the few broken moments of sleep he managed, he was never more than five minutes away. During the long days, he would sit by my bedside talking or reading to me, trying not to get in the way of all the tubes coming out of me. He read everything aloud. Letters, medical journals, scientific articles, work e-mails, books. The content didn't matter. He had read and heard that the only thing that mattered for me to feel safe, and maybe even wake up, was the sound of his voice.

Peter was given the phone number of a psychologist. Talking to a faceless stranger about the impending death of the person closest to you is a difficult task, but Peter needed answers. Above anything else he heard from the psychologist was that he would need to prepare himself for my death. And in the course of another conversation, a nurse indicated that he should think about whether or not to turn off the ventilator that was keeping me alive. Even if my brain was no longer working, she told him, and there was no prospect of it ever getting going again, there was still a chance that I could save someone else's life by donating my organs.

These were dark-blue times for Peter. There are many hours in a day and he had a lot of time to think and as he sat there next to me, in moments where he was unable to talk, he planned my funeral. We had never talked about what we wanted when the end came, and so he had to go on what he thought I would want.

There was, in fact, no doubt in Peter's mind that my ashes should be scattered in Cambridge. Some of our happiest years had been spent there, when the children were much younger and Peter and I were both working— he as a university researcher and me as a postdoc. We had spent three years immersing ourselves in the rhythm of this most traditional and historic of English towns. The children had all learned to speak English with a fluency they have to this day, and we had been drawn closer together as we explored the town and its surroundings. And so, Peter envisioned a beautiful ceremony by the River Cam, scattering my ashes on the gently flowing water, letting me be part of the place forever.

This was exactly what I would have wanted.

As the days went by and I remained in a coma, various causes for my sudden illness were eliminated. I was diagnosed with pneumococcal meningitis, a bacterial form of meningitis. *Streptococcus pneumoniae* is a special kind of sugar-coated bacteria that acts like a tiny armored vehicle destroying everything on its way through the human body. In most cases, it is caught by the spleen and the symptoms will be a mild cold. But in me, the bacteria seemed to have no barrier, sending toxins through my body. This ominous darkness spread everywhere, including into my brain, where multiple small blood clots exploded deep inside. It also caused a large hematoma, a swelling of blood that developed in the right side of my brain, which, if it continued to grow, would eventually extinguish the light in my mind. I would never again be myself.

My body had worked overtime to produce myoglobin, a protein that provides oxygen to keep us going for longer when performing. Too much myoglobin is not good. The muscles cannot handle it and release it in the body, where it produces a toxin compromising almost every organ. Usually the kidneys take care of the problem by flushing the extra myoglobin through the urine. But if there is too much, the kidneys give up. And if your kidneys give up, you stop producing urine, and all the bad things your body is perfectly adapted to get rid of start building up inside you.

All parts of my body were fighting each other. It was a battle with multiple enemies and no allies. My entire being had turned into one big myoglobin storage unit with more than four hundred times the level of the maximum normal range. If none of the other things that were happening were going to kill me, this certainly would.

The main focus was on saving my life, and every hour, every day during the first week was touch-and-go. But now knowing what it was, the doctors started to turn their attention to why this could have happened. During the many scans of my body, they discovered tiny calcified remains where my spleen should have been. Somehow, I had lived—undetected—without a spleen, my fortress against this particular bacterial infection, and this may well have been the key to why everything had gone so wrong.

Peter was by my side the entire time, keeping track of my treatment and any iota of change in my condition. He was also there to explain complicated medical terms, the technical details and multiple test results, and convey the doctors' messages to my parents and my sister, to my in-laws and his own sisters and, in a completely different and private way, to our children.

A week into my coma, Peter emailed our friends and colleagues, which resulted in an avalanche of love and support in every conceivable form: flowers, messages, poems, and letters. Even though I was unable to respond or understand, Peter and the children would read every single word to me, standing or sitting at my side. With so many people wanting to know what was going on and how I was doing, a spontaneous communication network was established. My family and closest friends and colleagues served as an important hub delivering Peter's messages. With little to do and only allowed brief visits to see me, they talked to each other, they called other family members and friends, and they let their worries and worst fears run free.

Privacy was not something of which I had the privilege. I was exposed and needed help in every possible way. Caring for me was about making my unconscious body as peaceful as possible and trying to prevent it from developing bedsores. It was also about showing consideration for my family and respect for me as a person. I was barely alive, but I wasn't dead yet. The nurses were gently covering up a horrible reality and trying to make me look presentable. Every day nurses washed me and made sure I was lying with my arms and legs at rest, though they couldn't do much else for my comfort, of course.

One nurse in particular liked to wash and comb my rapidly thinning hair. She even braided it. Others had different ways of making me look pretty, neat, and as close to normal as you can get when you are bloated, discolored and comatose. They took special care when the children came and made sure to cover my damaged body, especially my hands. My blackened fingers had started to dry up and wither.

About a week had passed when Victoria brought in a photo of me and put it next to my bed. Standing outside in the sun at a Cambridge college, huge purple and white flowers behind me, I had a big smile on my face. It was summer, and I radiated the happiness I was feeling at the time. And somehow this photograph, this one passing moment of my life that captured me then at my very essence, made a difference. Doctors and nurses started looking at it before they looked at me in bed. They talked about it, asked questions about it with whoever was with me, questions about where it was taken, what I was doing there, my work then, my work now.

From listening to the answers, they started to see a person, the woman whose life they were trying to save. The picture of me as a healthy, happy woman helped them to focus on me as a human being in the bloated, battered body in front of them. It was exactly what the nurse who braided my hair was doing, holding on to that person—even if that person, me, was nothing but a lump of flesh, fat, bones, and water.

In that picture I was Rikke.

THREE

Being

I have always been a fighter.

I am a mother, a wife, and a scientist. As a teenager I thought I would become a professional football player. I dreamed of becoming an artist. I have published scientific articles and books. I've curated exhibitions on science and art. I'm a cosmopolitan. I love traveling and have lived and worked in three different countries. I moved with my family from Cambridge, UK, to Cambridge, MA. I fell in love with California when living in Los Angeles. I cherish my Scandinavian heritage. I'm an Anglophile and yet feel comfortably American. It's weird, but it all makes sense, at least to me. I guess this is part of what makes us human: We are complex creatures, the composite result of our personal stories. In that way, I am no different from anybody else.

I was born on an island, in the same town as Hans Christian Andersen. Growing up on Funen gave you a sense of belonging and an identity. And if it didn't, people around you would soon remind you that it did. There was an almost tribal family system at work, making it difficult for outsiders to penetrate close-knit circles. There was a special island code you had to live by, part of which being that anything unfamiliar or foreign was subject to suspicion and scorn. Outsiders were scoffed at for talking or looking different, and for not enjoying traditional dishes, such as the smoked cheese or particular sugary brown cake. My family trusted the illiterate charlatan from the neighboring village, who would sell anything for a beer and a favor, more than they trusted an upright stranger.

My mother was a teenager when I was born and my father just twenty-one. With little education and a child to feed, they each had to work several jobs, and I was looked after by my aunt and my grandparents. As I grew older and started school, I loved going to the bakery where my aunt worked or playing with the children in my grandmother's street. It was safe and confined.

This was my world. Growing up in this community provided comfort and security. There was always someone to look after me. There was no need to go anywhere.

Many years before, my maternal grandmother had travelled far away, and as I played with the buttons in her "treasure" box she told me stories about the outside world. After the hardship of World War II, like many Scandinavians who had a hazy vision of America as a land of plenty and longed for something different, she had left Funen at twenty-two years old, ending up in the midwest on the plains of Nebraska, in a small town named Bassett.

My grandmother, the daughter of a nurse and a warden, was a practical young woman, used to working hard. She secured a job as a maid, her poor command of English of little consequence as she was a quick learner, happy, and determined to make it.

She liked her new country. In fact, she liked it so much, she overlooked the fact that legally, it was not her country. Technically, she was a Danish citizen living on a temporary immigrant visa. She didn't notice that her visa had expired and carried on working for many months, living her American life. Growing up in a Scandinavian country, with little knowledge of visas and immigration rules, she didn't even realize she was committing an offence by ignoring her expiry date. Eventually the local authorities got wind of her living in the town without authorization, and as she was unable to produce a valid visa, and her expired one had not even allowed her to work, she was sent back to Denmark, her American dream shattered. Permanently. By violating immigration laws, my grandmother was now a trespasser, an illegal alien, and the law came down hard on her. She would never be able to return.

The entire course of her life changed. She moved back to the town in which she was born, to become the lover of a married man.

That was my luck.

When I was three, my sister was born and shortly afterward my mother became very ill. We had to live with our grandparents for a while. My sister went to stay with my maternal grandparents, and I went to my father's parents. This was a decisive moment in my young life.

My father's mother worked at the local pharmacy selling over-the-counter pills. My grandfather was a hardworking, small-scale businessman. He owned a truck and drove around Denmark and northern Germany to pick up apples or sugar beets, or collect lumber, gathering odds and ends at farms, selling everything to the highest bidder, driving whatever anyone wanted anywhere. One of my earliest memories is going with him, being on the road before dawn, and singing our hearts out, enjoying the ride. I was five years old. My grandfather had been working pretty much since he was five himself, when he was sent out to work in the fields.

By the time he had children, he earned enough to send his sons to private school. To him, education was an investment in his children's future, but most of all it was an expression of love from a humble truck driver, who found it difficult to express his feelings verbally, to the people who mattered most in his life. I learned early on that education was important. My paternal grandparents were not exactly citizens of the world, but they taught me the value of diversity, the importance of tolerance and the benefits of knowledge and education.

My mother recovered and life went back to normal. But I continued to see my grandparents as much as possible. They had another, adventurous side to their lives. For a few months a year, my grandparents stepped out of their routine and managed a tiny shooting gallery at a local funfair. For me it was magical: the dance temple, the Miss Tanned Legs pageant, fairground stalls, large teddy bears, and all the ice cream and candy in the world. It was my favorite place.

Mostly I stayed around my grandparents at their stall or with my parents as they helped out, but one day I decided to explore. No one had seen me leave the stall, and when I didn't respond to my parents or grandparents calling me, panic set in. The atmosphere of the fair was mostly good-natured, but sometimes there was trouble with people who had drunk too much, and it was not a place for a little girl to be alone.

Other stall holders joined in the search, of which I knew nothing. I was with Svend, the biggest and friendliest man among all the tumblers and acrobats. He and I had developed a special bond, and as an undiscriminating child, I never saw how fierce and frightening he was to look at. While he drank beer, I drank the milk he had for me. Best of all was the strongly flavored, matured local cheese that I loved. We were sharing thick slices of it on dark rye bread when my parents found me. Oblivious to the commotion, my big buddy and I were happily eating away in our own little world.

My parents and grandparents were relieved to find me, of course. It turned out not to be a big deal after all. Everybody knew Svend. He was perfectly harmless, but my mother was left with a lingering worry about my free spirit that never really went away.

When I was eleven, my parents were able to buy a house and we moved from the city to a small village. As the new girl, my biggest worry was how I was going to fit in and to begin with, that wasn't easy, something any teenage girl can confirm. One day a classmate asked me along to football practice and that was what saved me. It turned out I had a knack for it and as she was their top player and because I was with her, I was drawn into the gravitational field of her popularity. I was in.

On the field, nothing else mattered to me but playing as hard as I could. There were no limits in how far I pushed myself; running, tackling, sliding in the mud, falling face down, gasping for air with hands at my sides, head down, my ponytail almost touching the ground. I loved it: the smell of grass, the sweat, the pain in sore muscles and chest from breathing the cold autumn air, the contact, the fouls and the pure pleasure of the perfect curved corner sailing past defenders and teammates, above the goal-keeper's hands to hit the net behind her.

Several times a week, I jumped on my bike to go to the neighboring town for training, and on the weekends, I took part in tournaments. This was my life. I improved rapidly, didn't do anything else in my spare time, and I soon came to see myself as a football player. And it paid off. My talent and killer instinct were spotted by a scout and my friend and I were both picked to train with the national youth squad.

My father was an avid football player and fan, and yet I lost count of the number of times I heard him say, "Girls can't play football!" How little that made sense to me: I was a girl, and I played football.

Maybe his refusal to accept my football hardened me in a good way. Standing in the rain, cold, tired, dirty, bruised, with a ripped shirt and two goals behind, I learned to bite down on the pain and fight, even though no one was watching.

Many years later, I used what I learned on the football field to take back my life. To push myself beyond limits. To never give up. It was the best training I could have for what was to come.

The first winter I was in university, age twenty, living away from home for the first time, my body collapsed. My kidneys had stopped working, my body bloated, and within two days I put on twenty pounds. I was examined by a number of specialists from oncologists to haematologists, subjected to a battery of tests and treatments, but no one could work out what was wrong. Nothing added up, and whatever treatment they tried only seemed to worsen my symptoms. My family stood around my bed crying, and the nurses looked at me with such tenderness, I could tell they thought I was dying.

The doctors were about to give up and let nature have its way. I heard what they said, but couldn't take it in.

How could anyone talk about giving up a life when the person was lying next door in a hospital bed hearing everything? A rheumatologist saved my life, diagnosing me with *systemic lupus erythematosus*, SLE, also known simply as lupus.

The reasons why SLE occurs are still not clearly understood. Presumably a combination of genetics and environmental factors triggers the illness, which makes the immune system attack healthy cells, tissues, and organs. This is what happened to me. My body turned against itself and was eating holes out of my kidneys. The daily ten-pound weight gain was all the excess fluid that could not be processed by my body and, with no way of being expelled, was being stored-up inside me. And that wasn't all. At the same time, my spleen started deteriorating, something that nobody noticed back then. I would only learn that almost twenty years later, when I woke up from a coma.

Once diagnosed, I was told that I would have to live with the condition for the rest of my life. I would have to take precautions and special measures to make sure I did not trigger further attacks caused by the dormant SLE, and I had to monitor any symptoms constantly. I had to make sure I got enough sleep, avoid stressful situations, and keep out of the sun. And as if this wasn't enough, I would also have to give up playing football. This was a big blow, but the doctor told me that my body was too weak and my bones and joints too fragile for a rough contact sport. I did not accept his verdict, but I kept quiet.

The medication worked, slowly but surely, and I recovered. But this was not the identity I had carved out for myself, and with my young body beaten up and swollen, and a mind in turmoil, I plunged into an existential abyss. What was to become of me?

I spent three months in the hospital. It was tough. For much of it, while recovering physically, I was trying to come to terms emotionally with what it would mean to live with a chronic disease. My independent adult life was only beginning, and I had already got a glimpse of the end. This was a tough lesson for a young woman. But with it, I grew stronger and I came to see, pretty early on, that there is never one single way in life and if this was my path, I would take it and meet the challenges along the way. It did me no good to think of myself as someone living with a disease. Having SLE was simply who I was. It did not make me more or less of that person. Some people need glasses, others a hearing aid. Some live with diabetes, others with asthma. I just had to live with this.

I started to make plans for the future—to go back to university. But lying there in my hospital bed, I realized that

I had to make a new beginning, something bold, to create a blank sheet for myself. I had to get off the island. Going to university in the first place was already quite a step for me. I had enrolled in a general science course, but I wanted more, or at least, I wanted something different. I decided to apply to study mathematics at a university in mainland Denmark. I received a letter of acceptance on my birthday. I couldn't have imagined a better present.

And like that, I left. My mum worried and my dad didn't see the point of moving so far away. They agreed it was like the other side of the planet. In reality, it was two hours in a car. I felt great.

I had been the first person in my family ever to graduate with a high school diploma, and I'd felt the entire world was open to me. By going to university, I had also taken steps no other member of my family had ever taken. But it wasn't easy. University was tough. It was an entirely new world. The people were different. The ways were different. The language was different. It changed me profoundly.

All my life I had felt slightly out of place. I belonged, certainly, but part of me was kept in a safe place where no one could gain access. As a child I never fully realized how different my academic aspirations were from everything in my working-class background. In my dreams I was reading, studying, and traveling. This was my secret, my personal hiding place, where I would run when things around me got overwhelmingly normal and I didn't fit in. This was my sanctuary, hidden away from family circles. A place of understanding, encouragement, empathy, and adventure. It was also a lonely place.

Going to university made me realize for the first time that I could begin sharing this part of me with others. I met like-minded people and gradually let them in. I learned that being normal was always a matter of context, and, adapting to my new surroundings, to the people and the competitive environment of academic life, I began to feel as though I could fit in. There were days, however, when I thought I would never be able to make it and, like many others trying to break the glass ceiling, that my background, my upbringing, was working against me.

Everybody at university comes from somewhere. Everybody has a story. Some people are born into academia and come with strong family traditions. They float elegantly in the air like circus artists on the trapeze, weightless, showing no signs of stress. For the rest of us, it is more difficult. My first years were a hard battle and a tough test. But I made it and continued through my graduate studies. I met Peter and fell in love. He was different from any other person I had met, generous, knowledgeable, always putting others before himself, a safe place in a storm. He saw me for who I am and embraced me as I was. The better I got to know him, the more I wanted from life. Once again, my world grew bigger. Best of all, we became a family. I graduated, got a job, we bought a house. By the time our youngest, Daniel, was born, I was thirty. Life was great, but again I realized I wanted more.

A wild scheme was planned. I had been working for a few years after my MSc in mathematics and art history, and had published a series of articles and a book, when I realized that if I wanted to continue with an academic career, I had to get a PhD. I pooled together what I had done already and made an ambitious plan to complete the degree program within a year. An evaluation committee decided it would be difficult, but possible. I got the grant and started to work like mad.

Peter and I made a pact.

"This is your year," he said. "You will write your thesis, I'll take care of the kids and everything else."

Johan and Victoria supported the plan. Daniel was still a toddler. He was OK with everything.

By the end of the year I was beginning to feel the full weight of it. I hadn't taken any break from my studies; no weekends off, no holidays. I was single-minded and determined, working toward my goal, stretching myself, pushing myself to my limits. It was a brutal regime, and while Peter took care of the children and they tried their best to understand that I had to work, even if they wanted to play, it wasn't entirely uncomplicated and they were all looking forward to the end of it.

That was a very gray Christmas. Peter and Victoria did their best to decorate the house and bring in some Christmas cheer, but it was all pretty lackluster. I didn't notice. I was too busy writing. Christmas morning came and I was still at it. On New Year's Eve at half past seven, we drove to the university, all five of us, and printed the entire thing. I was done. Completely done and utterly exhausted. And as I looked up after all those months of hard work, I saw my children as their mother, and not as the stressed-out doctoral student I had become. I made sure that we celebrated the coming of the New Year in style.

A few days later, when I had officially handed in my thesis, we left for a two-week holiday in the Canary Islands. It was warm and sunny, relaxing and restorative. Walking toward the beach, down the steps carved into the rocks, Victoria held my arm with a firm grip as we walked together, like one.

"I really like it when you are not writing your thesis. Now we can finally count the steps we climb again," she said.

And we did. I was badly needed. It had been tough on everyone. I had been missed and now I could finally be a mother again.

Living with SLE, I had very few side effects compared to the average SLE patient. However, one late-autumn morning in 2011, I had this overwhelming sensation that pouring tea from the teapot in front of me was insurmountable. For the past three months, I had experienced severe pain in my joints, in my hands and arms in particular. Not to be thwarted, I thought about various ways to overcome this challenge. What if I moved our teacups next to the teapot? Or if I tilted the teapot without actually lifting it? That would work. But it didn't. I couldn't pour the tea and in the end, I had to ask Peter to do it. I was devastated. Was this merely the beginning of what was to come? A year or two from now, would I have difficulty lifting my books, tying my shoes, or even combing my hair?

As Peter watched me struggling, he told me about a colleague he had met recently at a conference. She was a vegan. She had lived with severe pain in her joints every day until she changed her diet, avoiding all animal protein. Now her pain was gone. Completely.

Peter had mentioned me to her, how I had not been able to lift even small things for the past few months, particularly in the morning. He never asked specifically about her medical condition. It could have been lupus arthritis or a crueler rheumatoid arthritis, which causes severe destruction of the joints and in many cases disables you through deformities of hands and feet. She was a scientist, a highly skeptical one it turned out, who did not jump on the bandwagon of dietary fads. She had done her research, read the literature and dismissed most of it. But the little empirical evidence in the few serious scientific studies she had found made becoming a vegan worth a shot, she thought. And it changed her life.

"Why don't we try it," said Peter, tirelessly trying to cheer me up. "I'll do all the cooking and will support you in any way I can."

That's my husband, always looking out for me, eternally supportive. But no. I wouldn't do it. If this special diet had any effect, science would already have told me. I was a skeptic.

I grew up eating meat every day. The most natural thing for me to do as a teenager coming home from school was to have a couple of slices of rye bread or white bread with pig's fat, fried onions and sausage or paste made from pork liver. Before I went to high school, I don't think I had even met a vegetarian. My parents used to order half a pig or half a cow for the freezer once or twice a year, providing us with protein for many months ahead. Admittedly, I had grown out of the need for pig's fat and pork liver paste a long time ago, but I still liked eating lamb, beef and cheese. Things I was not prepared to give up.

"Let's do it," Peter persisted. "Let's give it a try."

He suggested several dishes and asked me to go along with this idea for a couple of weeks. If I saw no difference, then we could revert to being carnivores. Thinking of it like that—an experiment that we could monitor—and seeing his deep care and concern, I agreed.

An interesting and challenging couple of weeks were ahead of us. Meat, butter, eggs, cheese, milk and traditional fillings for our sandwiches were replaced by soybeans, green beans, hummus, avocado, salad, and bread baked with olive oil and soy milk. On the morning of the fourth day, my joint pain had completely gone. I could lift anything I wanted. I could do anything. I was ready to take on the world anew. I got my hands back. I couldn't believe it.

As if to prove something to myself, I grabbed my sketch pad and started to draw. I had been drawing since childhood, and I loved it with a passion. I had been so afraid of losing it. I was so relieved, tears slipped down my cheeks. I still had it.

Some of my happiest childhood moments were spent drawing with my paternal grandfather. After he died, I continued to draw and paint on my own and as I got older it helped me, as it kept alive in me the cheerful, worry-free childhood days that I spent with him.

He was always so encouraging, and even when I attempted to draw difficult things, he had the right words for me. I particularly remember a horse.

"That's right," he told me. "Look at her legs, Rikke, and how she moves. Look at how she moves her muscles. She's a strong creature. Powerful. See if you can find that with your pencil. Feel it. Feel how strong she is. Be her, when you draw her and never give up, even though it sometimes feels impossible."

It was a lesson for life. He never gave me a hard time, but equally he never let me off the hook until I had really put some effort into it, and regardless of how my drawings turned out, he always told me how proud he was of me.

"There you go!" he said, as I showed him my horse that looked like a potato on stilts with a strawberry head. "*That's* what a *proper* horse looks like."

In my third year at university, I had taken a sabbatical from my scientific studies and enrolled in art school. I loved every single bit of it, and to have the opportunity to explore my creative potential felt great. In fact, I had liked it so much that I seriously considered applying to the Academy of Fine Arts, but I was still attracted to the sciences and so, combining my passions, I eventually graduated with a joint degree in science and art.

From a very young age, Daniel loved to express himself with pencil and paper, just like I did. In the months before I fell ill, I taught him to draw with perspective. And while I was still in a coma, unaware of anything going on around me, he drew a perfectly proportioned shark and hung it on the wall next to my bed. He wanted to show me that he now knew how to do the things I had taught him. He wanted me to be proud of him. He wanted me back. My youngest child was reaching out to me through our private language of art, his perfect shark an expression of love, even if he wasn't sure I would ever see it.

All my life I had learned to keep going, to give it everything I had, to never stop fighting until the final whistle blew. But now it was not up to me anymore. My adult life had been different from anyone else in my family. I had graduated from high school and university, I had a PhD in science and pursued an academic career in top universities around the world, and now I was even a vegan, something as alien as a Martian to my family. I was not supposed to end up here in a hospital bed, not yet forty.

I was supposed to live a long life. I was supposed to bring up my children and see them safely into adulthood. I was supposed to grow old with my husband. Now, none of that was certain.

FOUR

Blinking

I opened my eyes with great difficulty.

Everything was hazy, almost no light coming in. I tried to keep them open, but it was hard and it hurt. Peter was sitting next to me and telling me about the snow outside the window. It sounded beautiful. I loved the sound of his voice.

"Winter has come," he said.

The kids and their father loved the snow. I wanted to see it, wanted to tell them to go outside and play. But even though I could formulate those words and thoughts in my mind, I couldn't summon the power to speak. I could not move my head or my hands. I could feel tubes in my mouth, but no other part of me. Where was I? What had happened to me?

My alarm did not register with Peter, who continued talking about the snow. Couldn't he see that I was trying to reply, that I was trying as hard as I could to get his attention? I tried to shout, to whisper, to wave. But everything in me was locked.

I was getting really scared now. I was doing everything I could to communicate, but the only thing happening was a slight dilation of my pupils behind my barely open eyelids. Was this really all I could do? Peter finally stopped talking. He looked at me and as he realized that my eyes were half open, he stopped, took a deep breath and leaned in closely. I dozed off.

I don't know how long I was gone. I had no sense of time. When my eyes opened again, ever so little, the bright light felt like tiny shards of glass shooting straight through my irises, deep into my brain. The pain was almost unbearable. I wanted them to close. I just wanted peace.

"Rikke, you are in the hospital, in intensive care."

What was he talking about?

"You've had a bacterial infection and you've been in a coma. But now you're back," he said.

Later, I sensed that I had woken up surrounded by darkness. I tried to open my eyes, but I forgot how to do it. Should I push or pull my muscles? Was it like doing push-ups? Yes, that was it. I just had to put some effort into it. But there was nothing I could do. My eyes remained closed and it was difficult to keep focused. His voice became more a comforting sound than actual words that I could take in. Meaning dissipated. I slowly drifted away.

My eyes opened again, like they had a mind of their own. I could hear Peter talking to me. I wanted to tell him I felt safe by his side. But I couldn't speak or move a muscle. I could hear my voice shouting inside my head, and I wanted to scream. It was like the most horrifying claustrophobic nightmare, except I was awake. Maybe I was suffocating. My bed felt like a coffin. Perhaps everybody around me thought I was dead and they were about to bury me without giving me a chance to tell them that I was still alive. Was this, in fact, the end? I sank back into the darkness.

This happened over and over again. Each time Peter told me what had happened, I was swathed in confusion. I was disoriented; I didn't know why I couldn't move, why no one was reacting to my thoughts. I couldn't understand why I was unable to speak. I didn't know why my body wasn't obeying my orders.

The only thing I could do was to listen and watch and hope someone would notice that my eyes were slightly open and would guess what I was thinking.

There are no Hollywood moments in waking from a coma. When you imagine it, you think of someone waking up, asking, "What happened? What did I miss? What am I doing here?" But in real life, in real hospitals, waking up is a process, a fragmented jumble of impressions, lights, and sounds. It is painful and noisy, so the urge to close the world out forever becomes overwhelming. You don't want to wake up; you would rather shut it all out and go back to sleep. You aren't conscious the way you are when reading a book, watching a film, having dinner with your family, or taking care of things at work. You drift in and out of consciousness, and you can't control it.

What took me a few seconds before my coma could now take an entire day. Trying to remember my own name, for instance, even when I had just heard it; trying to remember what someone had only recently told me, that for a fleeting second I knew I should try to hang on to. Those were overwhelming challenges that completely drained me of energy, making me sink into a deep, hard, dreamless sleep for hours. I was operating on a different timescale and in a completely different environment.

It took a long while before my eyes opened fully and in the normal sense of the word. At first it wasn't a conscious act. It simply happened. I knew nothing of it and to my family it was all going painfully slowly. I had what the doctors called sunset eyes. My eyes did not close. They were nothing but tiny slits, barely open with only a downward gaze, letting me peek into a world I had not been a part of for ten days. Or rather, it was a chance for everyone else to look in, to see if there was anybody in there.

The initial sense of joy everybody felt from the first minute my eyes had started to open quickly chilled. The doctors warned Peter not to get his hopes up. Sunset eyes were typically seen in patients with severe brain damage after long-term coma. I might have some sort of awareness of things around me, but I would probably never be able to talk again, to have a normal conversation, to eat by myself, to do everyday tasks, or even to recognize him or any of our children again.

And if I ever did wake up from this, if I ever recognized my family, if I ever started talking, the chances were that I would be a different person. The kind of damage done to my brain was linked closely to personality. I might be aggressive, less loving. I might shout and cry, not knowing why. I probably wouldn't even recognize myself. And this was if things went really well.

Peter had seen the images from the many scans. He had seen the dark spots deep inside the center of my brain, and he had gone quiet as the circular grey area grew bigger on the right side, a definite sign of internal bleeding. Blood clots and bleeding at the same time. Not a good sign. Whichever way you looked at it, this was bleak, but Peter took it and filed it and then ignored it, as he saw what no one else could see: a tiny light in the dull darkness of my downward gaze. Maybe there was still hope I would find my way back.

My carers and family members quickly became used to my downward gaze. But then tiny changes began to happen. Peter realized that my eyes closed gently if he asked me to close them. Sometimes, briefly, he noticed that my eyes moved slightly toward the direction of the room from where he was talking. He felt hope growing inside his chest. He thought he could detect signs of fight in my downward-looking eyes; see the stubbornness, strength, and resilience that had been my calling card since I was young. He wanted to believe it. The whole family needed to believe it.

In the horror of the first few days, when no one knew whether I was going to live or die, Peter had been advised that, while the scientific evidence was inconclusive, some medical experts believed that people in a coma responded to familiar voices.

"You never know," one doctor said to Peter. "She might hear you and this could be the thing that makes her want to return."

Noticing the tiny reactions in me, Peter and the children now had something to do, something that could help them to keep sane and give them a sense of purpose. They could talk to me and watch for my reaction, monitor the movement in my eyes, make a contribution to my recovery. They had derived comfort in talking to me even in the absence of response or reaction, but from the moment I started the long process of waking up, there was a new impetus in their mission. Peter had read to me every day, using every waking hour, every break between check-ups, treatments and tests. When I was still in deep coma, he read me Jane Austen's *Pride and Prejudice*. I loved that book and knew many passages by heart. Perhaps, he thought, it would trigger my sleeping brain to listen to something familiar, something associated with happy memories. At least now he had reasons to believe that something would get through to me. The children were also enlivened by my progress and each afternoon or evening took turns reading out all the new letters, cards, stories, and poems that friends and colleagues had sent. They told me what happened at school, what the teachers said and what they had eaten for lunch. They asked me questions, they sang to me. All this created a bubble, an illusion of safety, an artificial haven, and a world in which you were talking to your mother and she was listening. Even if there was no response.

They were now living with hope. I was still oblivious to everything, except, every now and again, I instinctively sensed their presence.

For the children, life was now a process of constant adaptation. They were coping as well as possible in such a situation. One of Peter's two sisters had moved in to our house to be with them. She was pregnant and had a daughter Daniel's age. She lived a four-hour drive away, she had a busy life and an impending work deadline, but she came anyway and was doing her best to make life work. Daniel and Victoria went to school, but they were ghosts at their desks, waiting for the day to end so they could dash to the hospital to see me. Johan stayed at home with his aunt, his life in limbo, uncertain when he would return to school in Hong Kong.

During the first few weeks, my mother and sister came to the hospital every day, which entailed a two-hour drive each way. Peter's parents had also come every day and Peter's other sister as often as she could. But apart from making sure the children were OK, there had been little to do other than be there, standing, sitting, talking to each other, waiting outside my room. With the exception of Peter and the children, visits had been limited and brief.

No other family, friends, or colleagues were allowed. But their presence was visible. Messages full of love, hope and anxiety kept arriving in large numbers along with gifts, poems, and flowers. Lots of them. There were so many that the nurses didn't have time to change the water and at the rate flowers had been coming in, they didn't have enough vases for them either. Later, I was told that I set the record in Intensive Care for the volume of flowers in one room. I was missed and I was loved. In the early stages of waking up, I did not notice anything. But as the weeks turned into months on my long journey back to life, this helped me. I was finding that extra bit of strength I needed to go on, to continue, to fight. Feeling loved is the most potent healing power.

And yet, twelve days after arriving at the hospital, I still wasn't responding. Every now and again, my eyes would open or close slightly. But that was it. Perhaps the doctors were right. There was too much brain damage, and I would never truly wake up and be myself. Growing increasingly desperate to get any kind of reaction from me, Peter thought about what else he could do and decided to ask the doctors if a good friend of mine might visit. She and I used to share confidences at work, joys and frustrations, things we were proud of and things we would never talk to anybody else about. The doctors agreed to it and Peter called her. He tried to prepare her as best he could, gave her all the details on the phone, told her about the poor odds, how wrecked I was, the way my fingers looked, his desperation and pain.

Beyond the medical team, she was the first person outside our small family circle who was allowed into my room. She had thought she was ready, but seeing my totally wrecked body for the first time and all the technology that was keeping me alive, she was stunned.

In a soft voice, Peter told me who had come to visit. But there was no reaction, just as had been expected.

They stood next to my bed talking to each other. It is difficult to have a normal conversation in a hospital room when you have a person in a coma next to you. My eyes might have opened ever so slightly, but there was still no reaction, no movement at all. I didn't blink. I might as well still have had my eyes closed. They talked about all the letters and cards, the flowers, what people at work were saying and thinking. She shared how my colleagues were still in shock that something like this could happen to a young, healthy person, that those with young families themselves were hit especially hard; it so easily could have been them. She talked, too, about the silence that fell in the department when news about my current state was sent around, and how people got together to share their thoughts. Engaged in conversation, they no longer had their full attention on me.

This was when it happened.

I slowly opened my eyes and looked at them.

Peter grabbed her arm and with eyes fixed firmly on me, he nodded in my direction. They looked at me, both with an overwhelming sense of witnessing a miracle before their very eyes. My sunset eyes, the passive downward gaze that heralded a defunct brain, had changed.

I looked up, straight at them.

"Rikke! Can you see us?" said Peter, barely breathing.

It seemed like forever before anything happened, but eventually I blinked.

"Sweetheart! Do you understand what I am saying?" I blinked again.

"Do you see who is with me?"

I recognized both of them. I understood what they were saying, and I was able to answer his questions by blinking.

No one had hoped to see such a dramatic turn of events. This was the first sure sign that I had not lost all my cognitive abilities, that I was able to understand simple questions and that I could recognize people around me. Peter had hoped this was the case when he tried desperately to interpret my tiniest movement, but he had not wanted to instill false hope in the children and had kept it to himself. But now he finally had something to tell. After almost two weeks of terror, there was some good news at last.

The magical moment lasted for only a couple of minutes before I drifted back into my private darkness. They hugged with tears in their eyes, conscious not to disturb me, overpowered by what they had just witnessed. After that she left, and Peter went to call the children.

I had re-entered my life. The gradual process of putting myself together had begun.

When Peter came back in the afternoon, the nurses had raised my bed slightly. My gaze was fixed on him when he entered the hospital room. It was an exhausted gaze, but a decisive one that wiped me out. I soon fell back to sleep. I was hardly awake during the day. I would open my eyes for a few minutes and then sleep again for hours.

Over the next week, my mind moved constantly between a conscious and illusory state, trying to find answers and sense in my situation. I learned what had happened again and again. People around me were patient and methodical, going through details over and over. It didn't seem to make much of a difference. Each time I was surprised, confused, shocked, terrified, and saddened. They could not build on things they had already told me, but had to start all over again every time.

My short-term memory was completely gone. I couldn't remember from one moment to the next. This is perfectly normal following brain damage and long-term coma. You remember your first day of school, but what happened twenty minutes ago won't settle. But for me everything—past and present—was a blur and only a very few things made sense. I knew Peter and the children. But I had no idea who all those other people were, running around me, checking things, drawing blood, and talking to me.

As I woke each time, at first the only things I was aware of were humming sounds from machines, beeping noises, nurses and some doctors coming and going. But I was never sure. And then all the commotion, loud noises, shouts, banging doors, running, panic. I had no idea what I was doing there. I had no idea what had happened to me. No idea why I couldn't move a muscle, why I couldn't move my lips or blow air through my mouth. I had no idea why no sound was coming out and I didn't know what was going to happen. My body was my prison and my brain was no help. All I could do was lie there, totally still, helpless, waiting while the thoughts haunted me. Was this the end? Was this it? Was this now my life?

Peter kept telling me over and over again where I was, what had happened, and that I shouldn't be afraid of anything. But I was afraid. Every time I woke up and he wasn't there, I was terrified. Where was he? Why wasn't he there? Who were all these strangers? Why couldn't I move and talk? I often cried when I woke up alone. Tears were running from my eyes, with no sound, because I couldn't say anything. I was screaming on the inside for him to come. Nobody could hear me. Nobody could understand. I was trapped, panicking, terrified, and losing control until he would return. He might have been to get something to eat or to catch a few hours of sleep. He was never gone for long.

But a few minutes felt like forever.

I was locked inside my own body and had to come to terms with a different life. I would never be the same person again. I spent my days sleeping and thinking. These were the only two things I was still able to do on my own. I did a lot of thinking. Not the kind of deep philosophical thought about the meaning of life. It was fragmentary and personal, pieces of my past, flashes of memories, feelings, episodes, tiny moments of life with my family, friends, and colleagues making me sad, warm, or fuzzy. I was grasping for scraps left over in a brain battered from scores of blood clots and cerebral hemorrhage.

I was fighting for what was left of me, trying to keep myself intact. I was hoping still to be a bit of the person I was ever so slowly beginning to remember, stuck in my hospital bed with only two options of either opening or closing my eyes. My life was a puzzle and I was trying to put it back together, but a lot of the pieces were missing, and many of them, it seemed, were lost forever.

It took me weeks before I began to understand what had happened to me. I had lost my memories, my bearings, and my sense of self. I could not move, I could not speak. Even when I tried as hard as I could, I had no contact with my hands or my feet, my arms or my legs. I was unable to shake my head.

Apart from sleeping and thinking, the only other thing I could do was to blink. This became my link to the world. A nurse suggested using my ability to blink as a mode of communication. The code was easy; even I could remember it. One blink for no. Two for yes. I guess she figured that the likely answer to most questions was no.

This changed everything for me. I couldn't initiate a conversation or ask any questions. But I could participate, I could make a contribution, and if people asked the right questions, I could even have things my way. The trick was to get them to do it.

I needed help, and I needed a tool. This was how the spelling board entered my life. It was new to me, but to the medical staff working with patients who are paralyzed, it's a standard device and was brought to me now that I was able to communicate with the world. It is the simplest thing: the alphabet on a piece of cardboard. But it was just what I needed to let the world know what I was thinking.

Using it was no easy task, however. First, I had to get the attention of whoever was in my room if I wanted to say something. How do you do that if the only thing you have to communicate with is your eyes? I tried looking in the direction of the spelling board or looking away, when people looked at me, and then quickly looking over to where the board was supposed to be. I needed to know where it was. Sometimes it had been moved by a nurse tidying up, or by Peter, who didn't think it of particular importance where it was, as long as he knew. But I had to know. This was my only lifeline to communicating. This was my first step in interacting with the world again, and I had to know where the board was, so I could make people pick it up.

When they finally did, I had to follow someone's finger moving steadily from left to right, row after row, not blinking until it reached the particular letter I wanted. I had to watch very carefully and did my very best. But even in super-annoying slow-motion, fingers often went too fast. And I wanted to say so many things at once, we missed letters again and again. Either I blinked too slowly or the person trying to read me missed a beat. How do you signal if you have to go back or start over when the only thing you can do is blink? The answer is, you can't. Especially not with a wobbly short-term memory and severely deteriorating eyesight from scarred tissue.

So, when I didn't give the signal in time or the speller sitting next to me didn't pick it up, we had to start from the top again. Repetition. Reiteration. Reprise. It was wearing me down. But then again, so was everything else. And as with everything else, I just had to carry on.

Slowly, too, I began to make tiny steps of physical progress. Not every day and not things that most people would even recognize. I started to feel the pain everywhere in my body; I felt my own discomfort. My physical needs were simple: my nose itched or my arm hurt from lying in an uncomfortable position, sometimes for hours without anyone noticing. Imagine for a minute you have an itch on your back at exactly that point you are unable to reach yourself and nobody jumps in to help you. It doesn't go away, no matter how long you wait. And there is nothing else you can do. You have a constant itch and can only hope something will happen. It might take half an hour; it might take two hours.

Then suddenly someone turns your body over, not paying any attention to your itch, and in the process, gets your arm stuck in an awkward position that immediately starts to hurt. The person doesn't help you, and you cannot even communicate that you need help. You lie there for another couple of hours until somebody else comes along and starts drawing blood from your exhausted veins, oblivious to what you are going through. The relief of one pain was always the beginning of another and I remember thinking: This is now my life. I'm locked in and utterly dependent upon people, entirely at their mercy, and mostly as they come and go, they are not even aware of it. And I have to live with that.

My lips were dried up and I couldn't moisturize them. It was painful, but I summoned everything I had left within me and eventually, after several days, I was able to move my lips ever so slightly. Unwittingly, this was a breakthrough in communication, and my family began to lip read. I was using only the simplest words: yes, no, and hello. Peter quickly learned to mouth-read "never mind." This was my longest sentence. Hardly anything to impress anyone, but a huge step for me.

Most of the time, mouthing a few words or using the spelling board was really not worth it. I was fighting too much already, and I couldn't afford the energy solely to tell Peter or the children that I was glad to see them. The children rarely used the spelling board. They mostly sat close to me, sometimes leaning in and sometimes guessing what I was trying to say. I struggled trying to remember people and what my children were telling me. Much to Victoria's alarm, I appeared to have no recollection whatsoever of our cats. She told a story about how one of the cats was playing with a bird in our conservatory. Somehow I must have looked surprised and puzzled. Knowing how much I loved them and what a central part of our family life they were, she worried about how much more I might have forgotten.

Paying close attention to every little detail and word uttered about me, she collected and analyzed it all. When she reached a state of panic, she asked Peter if I was going to get my memory back and be able to remember our lives together. He told her that eventually everything would return to my memory. But he had no idea if that would be the case and in fact, he didn't think it would. I now inhabited a parallel world, and one fine day, if everything continued to exceed medical expectations, it might align itself to the world everybody else was living in.

Typically, long-term patients in an intensive care unit suffer beyond the initial illness that brought them there. Their minds begin to play tricks on them and this happened to me. Apart from staying alive, my main job was to keep myself sane.

Sometimes, the repetitive cycles of being told what had happened to me brought tears to my eyes. I had no control over this. It was like my body remembered how to react to sad things. Every single time it was a shock to me and because my mind was a slippery slate, it washed meaning away as soon as I closed my eyes. I forgot and the next time Peter told me what had happened, it was new to me again. It was devastating for him to watch the same reaction of grief and surprise in my face over and over again. He was told the pattern was normal given the circumstances, but he couldn't escape the grim thought that maybe the damage to my brain was indeed as bad as the doctors had predicted.

In my head, I started coming up with my own explanations about what had happened to me. Suddenly I thought I had the answer. We had been in an accident. A violent and terrible car crash in which Peter and the children had emerged miraculously unscathed, but in which I had taken the full force. And here I was. Locked in my bed for the rest of my life. Or: I had lost the twins we were expecting. I thought I could see it in Peter's eyes that he knew it, too. But it was all right, I wanted to reassure him. We had survived storms before and we would get through this as well. Forcing dream-like states upon my consciousness, everything felt real. It was difficult for me to think straight, to pay attention, to understand what was going on around me. I saw and heard things that weren't there, and I was frightened by my thoughts.

And of course, I was wrong. None of what I imagined had happened. No splintering of flesh and bones as our car crashed, no twins. I had not been driving. I wasn't pregnant. My brain was simply searching for likely scenarios that had put me in the hospital. Venturing on the longest spelling journey so far, I managed to get through the combination of letters, "car crash," "twins," "lost them." At first Peter was confused, but he saw the panic building in me, so he took his time and through a long series of his questions and my blinking yes or no, he finally got it.

"None of that is real," he said, trying to comfort me. "You are imagining things. But it's OK, sweetheart. You will be all right. You don't have to worry about anything. I am here to take care of you."

Diving in past the tubes and wires, he did his best to hold me and, for the first time since my illness had separated us, I began to get a firmer hold of my situation. Maybe there was something in the memory of his touch that unlocked my memory of who I was. Maybe that caring, compassionate, most loving of gestures allowed me to remember who I was. I never asked about the imaginary car accident or miscarried twins again.

My body was still in a terrible state. The orthopedic surgeon had been to see me early on when I was unconscious, and as the bacteria continued to invade my body, he had made the grim assessment that if I survived, which he doubted, he would have to remove my hands from the wrist up, along with my nose, some of my face, and several of my toes. After seeing me again, he was more optimistic.

"I'm glad we waited," he said to Peter. "Five years ago, we would have cut off the dark red and black areas as quickly as possible to prevent gangrene from spreading."

Peter had got used to this blunt hospital talk. Nothing surprised him anymore and nothing shocked him. He took in the information and thought about how to communicate it in a gentler way to family members. The blackness of my limbs was slowly retreating as my body fought back, trying to recover lost parts.

"New research shows that the longer we wait, the more tissue we save," the surgeon continued. "We'll see how much it withdraws. So far, the prospects are good."

He had seen it all, including a patient who had part of his face, his hands, genitals and most of his legs removed. But, as he said cheerfully, that patient was happy. He was alive, and he really shouldn't be.

A few days later, looking at the doctor sitting in front of me, I was not sure if I had blacked out of a conversation again. It sounded like I had missed something important. I knew her. She was one of the intensive care doctors responsible for my treatment. I wondered what she was going on about.

"We wait until they fall off by themselves," she said. "As the surgeon explained a couple of days ago, the gangrene will eventually stabilize; your fingers will dry up and break off. The surgeon will tell you in detail how it works."

My eyes widened. Was she talking about *my* fingers? I had just woken up and was mostly concerned about dozing off again. My mind was still playing tricks on me. I had to remind myself where I was every time I opened my eyes. I summoned everything in order to concentrate and take in what she was telling me.

I couldn't believe what I was hearing: I was going to wait and watch *as my fingers fell off*? In that moment I realized that I was a passenger in my own life, no longer calling the shots, and that I was not in control. I would never run my fingers through my hair again, never snap my fingers to a catchy tune, never learn how to play the piano, never draw again. And I would never feel my children's faces through my fingertips.

I looked at Peter and blinked.

Once.

FIVE

Breathing

The day I learned I was losing my fingers, the doctors took my air away. I had been breathing through a machine every day at the hospital. With every muscle paralyzed, I couldn't inhale. My ventilator was doing it for me. Air was entering through a tube in my mouth and going all the way down into my lungs. The rhythmic sound of the ventilator added to the mosaic of sounds of the hospital, like an external heartbeat. It felt safe. But now my air machine was beginning to give me problems.

Wounds where the tube entered my mouth would not heal. My lips had built up black layers of coagulated blood, too fragile to clean. There were a lot of reasons why my coagulation system didn't work already. To prevent further blood clots in my body and brain, I had been put on blood thinners. But this had to be carefully balanced. One of the ways *Streptococcus pneumoniae* destroys the body is by making blood vessels porous, so if my blood became too thin, it could start flowing freely in my body, and then I would die from internal bleeding. To prevent this, I was kept on a complicated medical cocktail.

I was growing used to the plastic in my mouth. It gave me a sense of purpose. My teeth grinded against it in my sleep. When the nurses repositioned it, taping it down to keep it in place, I fought against it—silently and secretly—raking the depths of my battered brain to activate neurons so that I could move a few muscles in my mouth to push the tube, even by a millimeter. It was one of the only things I had control over and I badly needed to be in command of it. My mouth was full of sores going all the way down my throat. It hurt. Everything did. I couldn't keep my lips naturally moist, even if I wanted to. The high dosage of medication added to that, causing my lips to crack and preventing the sores from healing.

I was also unable to close my mouth, which exposed my teeth day and night, and meant that they completely dried up, eerily white and stained with black specks of hardened, sickly blood. They were impossible to clean, because of the tube from my ventilator and the risk that brushing them would cause my gums to bleed. The tube without which I couldn't live was making matters worse. To this day, my teeth are sensitive to breathing, and I try not to talk outdoors in winter.

But little by little I was gaining ground. Now, when I woke up, even though it might still take a while, I knew where I was. But my identity was still fragile: shaky in the brief moments between opening and closing my eyes. I was still so very tired and every time I closed my eyes, I didn't know if I would ever open them again. But if I could remember I had closed them when I opened them, I was winning. Remembering was control.

I could not extend that control to my breathing and needed my ventilator. Having the tube taken out of my mouth required a minor surgical procedure, the doctors assured me, and inserting a tracheostomy into my windpipe, a run-of-the-mill occurrence in an intensive care unit. Peter told me how great it would be not to have a tube down my throat, perhaps even to be able to close my mouth. "So," he said, "what do you think? Shall I tell them to go ahead?"

I blinked twice for yes.

I was taken to the operation room. Things happened faster than I had anticipated. I wanted to tell Peter that I needed time to prepare myself, but I didn't manage to get any signals through to him. In a few minutes, I was out and a surgeon cut my throat.

By the end of the procedure I was fitted with what, in technical terms, is a tracheostomy valve. Basically, it is a plastic tap. It left an open hole into my windpipe. Instead of the tube coming from my mouth to the ventilator, it now came from my throat.

I woke up in the middle of the night, drugged, disoriented, and full of pain, all the old terrors flooding my mind. I had forgotten everything; everything frightened me. I tried calling for Peter, I tried to pull myself up in the bed. But I couldn't hear my own voice, and I couldn't get my body to move an inch. I thought that everyone had gone and I was alone on the planet, that I was the last human left and there was nothing for me to do but to die.

The nurses working the night shift sensed my distress and ran to get Peter. I recognized him the minute I saw him and immediately relaxed.

"Hey, honey," he said, trying to hide how concerned he was. "They tell me everything went well and it won't be long before you should start feeling a bit of progress."

What on earth was he talking about? I was utterly confused.

My body had closed down as soon as the anesthesia had kicked in during the surgery and my brain was following its now-familiar pattern. It was as if I had been switched off again and was now reawakening from my deep coma.

My short-term memory had shut down once more. The tiny glimpse of hope from making a connection was quickly fading. Over the following days, Peter had to calm me down and explain what had happened over and over again. I became scared of falling asleep, afraid that I would never wake up, though I couldn't explain my fears on anything other than a superficial level of exhaustedly spelling out words.

Peter was devoting every waking moment to me. He was either sitting by my side, reading or talking to me, or he was gathering information, reading all the scientific literature he could get his hands on. Peter and I lived a life buzzing with science. At home we talked all the time about new discoveries and medical breakthroughs. We studied the facts, scrutinized details, and weighed the evidence before making any conclusions. Now, Peter was learning about septic shock and multi-organ failure. He was reading up on the latest research on long-term coma, SLE, thrombosis, spleen calcification and all the complications following from all this combined. It was his coping strategy. To be prepared, to be there when I needed him. And to be able to communicate even the harshest truths to our children, our parents, the rest of our family, and our friends.

He wanted to be on top of things, but he never really was. Just as the doctors weren't. He tried, though, and in all his grief, it helped. Peter was always focused, always present, even though the long days and short nights were taking their toll. He wasn't eating, he wasn't sleeping, and he was getting paler and paler. He knew the odds. He knew what the doctors were talking about, and they took him in as an equal. They started to have a real conversation. No sugarcoating and no nonsense. Because Peter is who he is, this was what worked for him. And because it worked for him, it worked for our children. It worked for me.

When he held my hand after my surgery, I couldn't hold his. I needed him. I could not figure out how to tell him, and it was overwhelming me. My body ached for him. I wanted him to hug me, to take me in his arms and carry me away to a time and a place where we could do whatever we wanted. It was as if my brain was calling up every one of its nerve endings. I concentrated hard, putting all of my energy into my face. Nobody else would have noticed, but when I almost invisibly puckered up my cracked lips to get a goodnight kiss, Peter did. Maneuvering in between tubes and wires full of air, food, blood and medication, he found a way. Our first kiss. An uncomfortable, awkward, but completely wonderful, kiss.

In the days after the surgery, everything remained hazy and the noises around me were indistinguishable. But slowly I began to remember people and what had happened. Change could come in the course of a single day. One afternoon, I could suddenly follow the nurses' instructions to open my mouth or close my eyes when they washed me, brushed my teeth, or combed my hair. In the morning, I hadn't been able to do any of that. Things were getting better and I embraced it all. I wanted to take every single step, as long as it was taking me somewhere else, away from this place.

The first direct result of the operation was that I was able to get air more freely and I was no longer feeling the constant pain of the tube cutting deep wounds in my mouth. The ventilator was still breathing for me, but one of the nurses told me, "It won't be long until you can start breathing by yourself. Bit by bit, Rikke. In fact, we are going to try it out later today."

What was she talking about? Had a doctor agreed to this? What happened if it didn't work and they'd turned off the machine? Would I die? Questions and panic were building inside me. I desperately did not want them to turn it off. I had no faith in being able to breathe by myself.

And yet I couldn't wait.

There was another huge difference, too. After thirteen long, bleak days, Peter and the children could see my face. Not the face of white plastic tubes and adhesive bandages to keep it all in place, but a human face. There I was. They saw me for the first time since I left the house, the face they knew so well and could read better than any book. To anyone else I was still a horrifying sight, but to Peter and my children, to my mum and my sister, who were still only allowed to see me sporadically, it was a sign that I might be returning to them.

Another day went by before they risked taking me off the machine. For the first time in two weeks I was now, suddenly, supposed to breathe by myself. I was scared out of my senses. I was trying to remember how to do it. I had learned to breathe within the first ten seconds of being born and I had never had to think about how to do it. Pulling air into my lungs, pushing it out again, regulated by centers in my brain. It happened automatically. Now, lying here, unable to do anything for myself, how could I be sure that the rest of my body hadn't suffered from amnesia the way my brain had? How could I be sure my body was going to do what it was supposed to do, when it couldn't figure out anything else?

"OK, Rikke, let's get on with it," the nurse said.

There was no doctor present, which alarmed me. Peter was standing by my bed trying to look confident, but was clearly not very comfortable.

I blinked once, but the nurse ignored me.

Within seconds, I was off the ventilator. It lasted less than two minutes. I would like to say it felt good, but the truth is, I felt as if I was going to die. I was pining for air, and my body was imploding from within. I wanted to scream that I needed the machine back on. There was no air coming through my mouth; it was all blowing straight through the open hole in my throat. Air was simply leaving my body as panic rose and darkness closed in on me. I was sure I'd lose consciousness and who knew what else. In a history of bad ideas, this felt like the worst.

After what seemed like forever, I was back on my beloved oxygen. I relaxed. I never ever wanted to breathe without my ventilator.

I hated it, but I knew I had to persevere. There was no going back. At first it was just a few times a day and not for very long. Each time was equally painful and frightening. I felt like a punctured tire.

Peter was always there, encouraging me—"You're doing brilliantly!"—but he was unable to hear my internal screams.

I didn't even notice when I finally breathed for myself.

"Sweetheart! You're breathing! You're doing it!" Peter and the nurse were keeping a close eye on the monitors.

I heard them, but I couldn't feel what they were telling me. It was bizarre: the oxygen levels in my blood were dropping, I was suffocating—and yet they were celebrating. The hose was put back on and I was soon within the normal saturation range. Somehow, apparently, I had started absorbing oxygen from the air around me, and this meant that for a few seconds, technically, I had been breathing. I wasn't very good at it. But suddenly I understood what the word meant. Even if it had been the hardest thing I had ever done, I had been breathing, on my own.

And the world changed again.

The next step was to fit a small device onto the tracheostomy sticking out of my throat, which would allow me to speak. I found that hard to believe. A valve would force air past my vocal cords, which would theoretically let me produce sound. This is the very foundation of speech. With no air coming through, there is no sound. I was desperate to try.

"Everything looks fine and works properly. You should be able to say something anytime now," a nurse told me. "Patients are often rather good at it."

OK, I thought to myself. If other people can do it, I can. Without thinking about actually what to say, I opened my mouth.

No sound. I tried again. Still, no sound.

This was not going the way I wanted. I started coughing up congealed blood that had been sitting in my throat. Still, I couldn't say a thing.

"You shouldn't worry about it, Rikke. This is also perfectly normal," said the nurse. "It will come."

I had hoped so much to be able to speak. The medical staff rarely used the spelling board. Only Peter and I spelled out longer conversations. To everybody else, mostly, I was answering questions by blinking for yes or no. I wanted more, I wanted to participate so badly. I wanted my voice to be heard. But I did not speak that afternoon.

Lying alone with my thoughts, I realized how much becoming a mother had changed me. My perspective had altered, and I'd learned to appreciate there was something bigger and more important in the world than myself, someone to take care of and protect. To this day, I will never be able to describe the pain I felt, unable to touch or talk to my children. It went far beyond the physical. I wanted to protect them, shield them from the pain they were feeling. I was trying desperately to express my affection for them, to let them know how much I cared about them and that I was still there for them. But how could I do that by just blinking? I missed them. All the pain in my body didn't touch the agony of not being able to give them a hug or stroke their hair.

Daniel told Peter that he was afraid I would never come home again, and that life had changed forever. At eight, he was preparing to live without his mother. But in all those months while I was away from home, he never told me how he felt. He kept up appearances for my sake, to protect me, who should have been protecting him.

The children came to see me every day, in the afternoon or in the evening. While I lay in bed, they sat around me, chatting, doing their homework, reading, sometimes singing—anything to keep their constant pain at bay. Part of their daily ritual was getting something to eat at the hospital cafeteria. Everybody working there soon got to know them. They knew what was going on, even if they didn't know me. Peter saw it in their eyes, the tiny nods, the small gestures of an extra scoop of pudding or a little treat. Sometimes when they came back after their meal, they were chatty. In this grim setting, any distraction was an adventure. But it only lasted for so long before the harsh realities hit again, and silence fell upon our tiny flock.

After two full weeks I was stable enough for Peter to be able to go home. He had been living at the hospital, never leaving, never more than a few minutes away from me. His room was needed by someone in greater need than him. Peter's pregnant sister would be able to go home, and the children, who desperately needed their father, would be reunited with him.

He had gone through the worst time of his life over these past couple of weeks, through unimaginable scenarios filled with disbelief and pain beyond words. All that time he'd had to be strong, for me and everyone around me. When he returned to our house, he had to re-enter life outside the closed environment of the hospital and be strong again for the children.

Victoria was hugely relieved by this turn of events. With her father out of the house, she had assumed a greater responsibility at home. With grandparents, aunts, and everybody else around her deep in their own grief, it was sometimes hard to appreciate her needs. She needed her father to let her be a little girl again.

Peter brought safety and comfort back home. He talked with the children, laughed with them, made dinner and, that evening, tucked them in, one after the other, none of them too old for such tenderness.

But then he collapsed. He broke down, the weight of grief pushing him to the floor by the radiator in our living room. For the first time since the ambulance left with my dying body, he cried. He could still hear the panic of the paramedics, the syringe falling on the tiles. When we'd first got together, we had assured each other that neither of us would ever be alone again. But we were wrong. Now he was alone, and he was feeling the weight of it. Every last ounce. In addition to charting and documenting on paper what was happening to me, Peter had been photographing the equipment, medication, charts, and clinical journals as well as my room, the children, the flowers and cards. He was building a private photo archive for me, even detailing the stages of how I looked, every little fluctuation in my condition. In the beginning, he took what might have been the last pictures he would ever have of me. He wanted to hold on to me. He wanted to keep me. And then, as I began to recover, he wanted me to see the journey I had made. These photos were snapshots of our love.

There were no easy days, no routines, nothing I could simply tap into and relax. Everything tested my mental and physical limits. I had to be turned, lifted and moved every few hours to prevent bedsores. My body was still paralyzed, but with a tremendous effort and patience from therapists, I was beginning to connect with a few of its individual parts. It took three people to get me lifted from my bed and turned so I could sit up, though sitting wasn't really the right word. I was propped up like a bag of potatoes, unable to support myself. If any helpers had let me go, I would have fallen flat on the floor.

Every single time I was scared witless. What if one of them slipped or another wasn't paying attention and failed to give me proper support at the right moment? The only thing I could do was to watch as my body was moved around and hope that nothing happened. I couldn't even give a shout of warning. I was a helpless mute, a desperate passenger, while others tried to maintain my body by moving its parts. It had to be done if there was to be any hope whatsoever that I would ever stand a chance of one day moving on my own. It was nauseating and frightening. I hated it.

Sitting or having my arms moved, I was told, was the equivalent of my running a marathon every single day. It felt worse. I was still locked inside my body, unable to talk or move, getting all my nutrients and water through my veins. I was still utterly dependent on my ventilator, but the time I could manage without it and breathe on my own was gradually increasing.

I was showing few signs of improvement. I had been on dialysis since being admitted, as my kidneys had stopped working completely and couldn't clean my blood. Without dialysis, waste products would accumulate in my body and eventually become lethal. A tiny drop of urine in a bag was celebrated as if it was my birthday, and as I began showing slight progress, the doctors decided to take me off the machine for a short while. As with the breathing, my body had to be pushed to do it, but as my kidneys responded reasonably well, the length of time off dialysis also increased, even though every now and again I had to have my system cleaned properly and go back on the machine.

I was beginning to get used to spending nights on my own, though I was never really alone, as a nurse had been assigned to me twenty-four hours a day. Peter went home every evening to be with the children. We lived over an hour away from the hospital, so it was impossible for him to return once the children were asleep.

One evening I managed to get the nurse working the night shift to pick up the spelling board.

Together we meticulously pointed and blinked "P-e-t-e-r" on the board.

"Do you want to talk to him?" she asked. It was her first shift with me, but she was already sensitively attuned to my thoughts. "Do you want to talk to him on the telephone?"

Could I? No one else had ever suggested that. Peter always called before bed to get a status report, but only ever talked directly to the nurse on duty.

I blinked twice.

The nurse called him back and put him on speakerphone. Then she withdrew to give us privacy, but not before she had told my news to Peter.

"That's amazing!" I heard him say. "The nurse just told me what happened after I left today." Then he told me: The nurse had put on the simple one-way speaking valve on my tracheostomy for a few minutes earlier that evening. Air was allowed in but not out and I suddenly found myself able to blow air, ever so little, through my teeth, making a hardly audible and yet quite distinct F-sound.

"Your first real sound!" Peter said, enthusiastically. "That's fantastic!"

I knew immediately that he was disappointed not to have been there—as if he had missed seeing the first steps of one of our children—but at the same time, he was so full of joy celebrating this crucial breakthrough with me on the phone, and now I had made one sound, maybe I would make more tomorrow and in the days that followed.

"Good night, sweetheart. I'll see you tomorrow. Sleep well. I can't wait to tell the children."

I wish I could have said something in return. And as I was still struggling with my short-term memory, in that moment I actually had no recollection of my sensational F-sound. But Peter was making me feel proud nonetheless.

I closed my eyes. I was on a roll: I was breathing, I was peeing, and I could say F.

Time for me to get started on the rest of the alphabet.

SIX

Healing

A few steps forward were always followed by a few
steps back. My state of being was a constant, delicate
question of balance, and I could go downhill fast. The doctors and nurses took regular readings of my temperature,
blood pressure, saturation, heart rhythm and rate and on
top of that, anything else that could indicate change
within my body.

All sorts of things could be ascertained from the reading
of my blood, one of them the levels of C-reactive protein,
or CRP for short. Scientists studying *Streptococcus pneumoniae* discovered that patients like me suffering from
bacterial infections produced very high levels of CRP. It
has now become a general indicator of an infection and
is one of the best ways of keeping an eye on how the body

is coping with it. Ever so slowly, day by day, as the bacterial storm raging in my body calmed down, my CRP levels decreased. This was a clear sign of healing, but it was no reason to celebrate yet or be complacent. It took very little to knock me out of kilter and my levels would rise again.

I had grown used to the constant comings and goings, the different greetings and mannerisms of the medical staff who came to care for me in any one day. There were doctors, nurses, and therapists I had grown fond of: ten, maybe twenty people a day. From very early on, I could identify the nurse who took my blood from the sound of her cart. I heard her before I saw her. Sometimes I wondered if she was trying to keep out of sight. She was neither friendly nor unfriendly. After saying hello, she got to work. She had a job to do, and I was only one of many patients on her rounds.

My veins were getting increasingly difficult to draw blood from, so I had been fitted with a kind of tap straight into my vein. This made her job easier, as she did not have to bother me trying to pierce my skin in the attempt to tease anything from my exhausted veins. She could drain my blood while I was asleep and many times I did not even notice. She screwed small canisters onto the tap, one at a time, and I watched as they steadily filled up with deep-dark red blood. As my blood drained, she didn't talk to me, only got the next tube ready to screw on, and when she had finished, she left as quickly and efficiently as she could. She never spoke to Peter. She must have believed that most of the time relatives would rather be left in peace. It was better to be on the safe side and drift into anonymity, serving your function and nothing else, and leave quietly and unnoticed. Later I learned it was seen as a badge of honor by some of the medical staff to be invisible, never to get involved, to let healthcare professionals be an anonymous, well-functioning curing machine.

Three weeks after I was hospitalized, we got an explanation of why I couldn't move. I was diagnosed with critical illness polyneuropathy, CIP for short—a paralysis of the nerves that control muscles—which had caused a loss of movement or sensation in my body. It usually increases with the length of stay in intensive care and it raises the possibility of death. Doctors told us there was a 50 percent chance that it would pass, and I would be able to move again. This was splendid odds compared to earlier. I was still almost nothing but an oversized human cushion; however, I was making progress. Peter was encouraged. He told me that one day I might even be able to get around in a wheelchair. Hearing this, I decided to fortify myself mentally to make more progress, whatever it took.

I was more awake, more conscious, and ready to talk. I was using the speaking valve regularly. I had so much to say, so many questions, and an overwhelming urge to participate in life and conversations around me. But no words, not even a single syllable, came out. While I was still locked in a body that would not obey my simplest commands, I was sentenced to talk to myself. I was, though, now able to follow some of the activity and conversations that took place around me, especially among the nurses in attendance. Sometimes they talked about me, but mostly they talked to each other about what they had done over the weekend, what was happening in the hospital, on the news, in their lives. I had no choice but to listen. They weren't talking to me because of the damage to my brain; some assumed I couldn't follow what they were saying. Sometimes I found myself eagerly awaiting the next installment in a particular story, but often I learned to conserve my energy by not concentrating hard on everything being said, and anyway, I still slept most of the time.

Most people on my medical team talked to me, looking me in the eye when they explained things to me or talked about my family, the photographs next to my bed, all the letters and the flowers still pouring in. I had so much I couldn't say back. The spelling board was rarely in use, as it was exhausting for everyone involved. It took patience, time, and stamina and as I was gaining more control of my facial muscles, I was trying to use my eyes more to communicate. It was a real revelation to me how much effective communication could take place from merely looking another person in the eye. I was also beginning to mouth more words. My most often-used phrase was still "never mind," following minutes of trying to convey a message like "my hand hurts" or "I'm so happy to see you."

Peter's tenacity and patience was invaluable to me. He could tell that I was able to understand far more than others realized. He knew I was in there, that it was me and not a chronically distorted, brain-damaged version of me. He and I talked about the possible brain damage. Sometimes a conversation could take days, but he persisted in staying with me as I slowly spelled my way through questions about what had happened to my brain, organs, and hands, and what would happen to me in the future. I wanted to know everything, and Peter answered truthfully. One day, as he once again meticulously went through everything from the ambulance to me waking up in a paralyzed body with multi-organ failure, I was finally able to express my feelings in a single word. Peter read "horrible" from my silent lips.

"I know, sweetheart," he said gently. I closed my eyes. One Sunday morning when my family came to see me, Peter could tell that I was not feeling well. I had always tried to spare the children any further distress, but I had never been very good at hiding anything from Peter. He asked me how I had slept.

"Thinking," I mimed slowly and looked him deeply in his eyes. "I'm scared."

At night, the demons came.

Whatever was going on with me, Peter was always allowed into my room, to be by my side. It was clear that I was calmer and more attuned to what was going on around me if he was there. And while the medical and therapeutic staff got on with their work, he sometimes chatted to them, asking them questions or, as I was improving, answering their questions about my progress.

One morning, Peter was standing outside my room with a nurse, getting last night's updates. The signs were good. I had responded well to everything the previous day and throughout the night. I'd had a good night's sleep. The nurse on early morning duty had just finished getting me ready and had elevated my bed slightly. I was being dressed. The nurse suggested that Peter wait outside for a bit before coming in and seeing how much better I was.

As she talked, I tanked. My pulse and heart rhythm dropped drastically, my oxygen saturation plummeted, and I fainted. All of a sudden, the situation was one of panic. Doctors and nurses flocked around my bed in another life-saving effort. The nurse talking to Peter ran in, closing the door on him.

After lying on my back for several weeks in a row, gravity had kicked in. My left lung had partially collapsed, and my lungs were no longer inflated at full capacity. The mucus stuck in my deflated lung could cause a serious infection that would be difficult to control, a relatively common precursor to a fatal dose of pneumonia. I had barely survived one infection; I was most certainly not ready for another.

I couldn't get rid of saliva and spit. Lung specialists were rushed in to find a way of treating me urgently without worsening the fragile state I was in. Trying to let me breathe on my own had quickly turned into mortal danger, and I was put back on the ventilator. They hurriedly installed a different kind of valve in my throat from which they could draw fluid directly through the nozzle. A simple contraption for a delicate maneuver whereby a nurse uncorked my throat and stuck a long thin plastic tube into the hole all the way down into my lungs. Like a vacuum cleaner, my new machine sucked the blood and slime stuck in my lungs. The pain was excruciating.

I hated it. I was ready to sacrifice the lung they were trying to save. In attempting to remove the obstacles impeding my breathing, the plastic tube rummaged around in my delicate lung tissue, and it hurt so badly I could hardly stand it. It felt as if I was falling fast—not exactly back to square one, but close. I was weak, and I couldn't stand the pain and, to counter another infection, I was put on a complex blood dialysis lasting four hours, rinsing my blood for waste products while everything else burbled away.

Peter had to wait a full agonizing hour before anyone told him what was going on. By then I had already been fitted with my new valve, and attempts at sucking my lungs free and inflating the collapsed lung again were made. He had seen doctors and nurses run into my room, wearing serious expressions with no time to explain what was going on.

And I had no strength to tell him myself.

I felt for Peter being at the mercy of other people's concern. Being in an intensive care unit, he witnessed terrible despair and desolation, sometimes relief and hope. Later he told me that he learned to read the relatives of existing and new arrivals, how to manage their looks of concern as he came in to see me day after day; how to focus on fragments of hope or anguish communicated through passing looks and nods. He learned the tacit language of grief-stricken outsiders confined to waiting in hallways, while there was nothing for them to do. On the day my lung collapsed, he took in their compassion and under-standing. Theirs was a shared language of coping; the poetry of grief.

He also got to know many of the professionals who were caring for me, distinguishing among those who wanted to talk and those who didn't. There was the grumpy older doctor who brightened when he and Peter talked about the latest details of research on infectious diseases; the young doctor who'd seen so much but not enough; the skinny nurse on night duty who talked about going out clubbing but so often stayed on, lighting up the last hours of some patients in her care; the porter who loved art; the physical therapist who threw herself into her work with the same dedication as an Olympian coach. Peter was spending so much time in their company that this new cast of characters became familiar—not close, but near—as he gradually grew out of being an intensive care rookie.

My fever kept coming back, with new signs of infection. Antibiotics were administered carefully, intravenously, but despite a constant flow of medication, I was still incredibly sensitive, an easy target for the old infection to strike again and new ones to aim for. Even after three weeks in the ICU, the doctors were unclear as to exactly where my original infection had begun, though they thought they had narrowed it down to my lungs or my sinuses. A new group of medical experts conducted an ultrasound test confirming an abnormal accumulation of fluids in the sinuses and so, to prevent anything new from building up, I now had to have drainage tubes put up my nose. Effectively the tubes were made up of tiny microsuction pipes that were used to rinse my sinuses every day. Yet another piece of plastic, making it increasingly difficult to tell where my own body began and ended.

And it hurt. Before all of this happened to me, I would have said that it hurt like nothing else. Now it just hurt like everything else.

So did breathing off the ventilator. But I had to do it, as my life-supporting air machine was now a major contributing factor to my physical deterioration. I would never overcome the CIP that was paralyzing me if I did not start moving my body. The doctors had to find a way for me to activate the muscles controlling my breathing, if I ever hoped to be able to do it completely on my own. The most effective way of doing that was through a process of suffocation—by taking the air provided by my ventilator away and thus forcing my body to react. After my lung had collapsed I was more fragile, so it was more difficult to breathe unassisted. I felt as if I were drowning in air. But, as the doctors explained, breathing on my own was the only way to inflate my sticky lungs, glued together by blood and phlegm and sealed by gravity.

I hated it. I truly did. Like everything else at the hospital, it had now turned into something I would rather never see or feel again in my life. But I also knew there was no way around it and that for now, I was utterly dependent on the equipment and help that I loathed so much. The hospital was both my threat and my safety, the only place in the world I could survive. I would not last half a day on the outside.

Then there were good signs. My potassium levels were dropping, indicating that my kidneys had started working again, ever so slightly. Perhaps, if I recovered and was able to return home one day, I would not need lifelong dialysis. Even if I did, doctors had assured me I could still lead a rich life. I should have felt grateful for just surviving. I was and I wasn't—a mass of contradictions.

While my body was slowly healing, I was gaining ground in my mind. Just enough to realize how much was wrong with me and how terrifying it was to be confined to my bed, unable to participate in my children's lives. It was like a living hell not to be able to talk to them, or to laugh with them, or gently to wipe away their tears and tell them that everything was going to be all right. That their daily visits, and Peter's near-constant vigil, was what stopped my mind from descending into freefall.

As my mind became stronger, a new problem appeared. I started dreaming, but with that my conscious and unconscious mind began to merge. This was not a good thing. Being in a coma had, in some ways, been gratifying, as I'd been completely out of it. If I had been dreaming, I hadn't realized it and I certainly hadn't remembered anything. And since coming out of it, I had used everything within my grasp just to hold on to myself, to try to regain some control while awake. But now, I couldn't always work out whether I was asleep or awake, if I was experiencing a reality or dreaming my way through the moment. In short, it was getting increasingly difficult for me to distinguish between what I was thinking and dreaming, and what was actually happening.

I was getting delirious. This is completely normal for patients after emerging from a long-term coma, lying for days on end in intensive care. Ironically, a nurse had told Peter about this form of delirium by saying how extraordinary it was that I had no signs of it at all. She had spoken too soon. The next day, I became fixated on—and beyond outraged by—the belief that Peter had paid a therapist an exorbitant amount of money to give me a massage, but she never turned up. I was convinced she had just pocketed the money for a service never rendered; but this was not the only source of my outrage. I was also overwhelmed by the idea that she had been able to swindle me in Intensive Care. If there were thieves running around the ICU in a major hospital and nobody else noticed, then how could I ensure I was safe, that my children were safe when they came to visit me?

I had to tell the staff. I had to warn them. But then again, what if they were in on it? Could I really trust the doctors or the nurses or my therapists? And what about all the medication they were feeding me around the clock? What was the real reason I could no longer move or talk? Was I a prisoner? An experiment? As my delirium took hold, the familiar sounds lulling me to sleep were now threatening. The walls were closing in on me. The room started to turn and tilt. The ceiling dropped. Now the only thing I could hear was the sound of my own blood, like rhythmic mini-storms raging in my ears. I had to get out before they finally took me over. I was still in with a chance.

I needed to find out what we were going to do about the therapist, and how we could call her to account. It took me an entire day using the spelling board, mouthing, winking, sleeping, and waking up to tell Peter about the rogue masseuse running wild at the hospital. At first, he was utterly confused and had no idea what I was going on about. Then he realized the delirium was hindering my progress.

He was right. But it wasn't only the delirium. I was suffering from a constant fever, my sinuses were being brutally rinsed with saltwater, my lungs routinely vacuumed for blood and slime. My CRP was going up and down, indicating an infection that was proving difficult to get rid of. I was still operating on a faulty short-term memory. My life was now what I experienced when I looked around. Sometimes bits and pieces stuck for a few hours, like memory debris, but most often they slipped away again.

I was, however, gaining an understanding of how seriously ill I was and could grasp some of the consequences. As I was still unable to talk, I spent most of my waking hours scanning my room. Peter noticed that I was spending more and more time looking at my hands—my black and dried-up fingers that would never heal. Johan had seen this, too, and had asked his father about them; Peter explained what our oldest son had already guessed.

To protect Daniel and Victoria, the nurses had the habit of covering up my hands during visits. One day, the nurse forgot, and they saw. They didn't say anything to me, but as soon as they got back home, they bombarded their father with questions. He told them the truth—that it was likely my fingers were going to fall off. They all cried, Daniel and Victoria unable to stop. In an effort to comfort them, Peter prepared their favorite snacks and made a comforting pile of duvets in our bed. Eventually they all calmed down and fell asleep, a tangled family bundle. Despite all the progress I had made, our children now knew that some things would never be the same again.

I was not the only one who needed to heal.

SEVEN

Tilting

I had physical training and occupational therapy every day, even when I was still in a coma. Because I was completely paralyzed, I lost body mass fast. Muscle weakness had set in only a few days after I went into coma, and from that moment my body had started, and now continued, to wear away. This affected my blood circulation and breathing, which made me even more vulnerable and reduced my chances of full recovery. The only way of maintaining muscle mass and preventing serious side effects was to move or *be* moved.

Doing so required a team of specialists trained to shift my limbs gently without doing any damage. I was assigned a physiotherapist and an occupational therapist. My physio focused on general mobility and muscle strength, while my occupational therapist zoomed in on specific tasks such as grabbing or holding an object; though initially, all she could do was to massage the non-damaged parts of my hands and feet. For several weeks, I didn't participate actively in any of this. Everything was done *to* me, and even when I moved into a more conscious state, I was a passive observer. Peter wanted to help as much as he could and quickly became adept at lending a hand.

The first time I was maneuvered into a semi-upright position at the side of my bed was after three weeks of being admitted. It took a group of three professionals—and Peter—half an hour to get me up, hold me in a sitting position for ten seconds and then lower me down, back into bed. It was a complicated procedure involving a transfer sheet and a lift, a bit like a large robotic arm picking me up in a carrier bag. These maneuvers were followed by several hours of exhausted sleep. To an outsider, ten seconds of sitting up would have barely registered as progress, but for me, every second of being upright was like climbing a mountain. After a week, to the delight of my therapists, I had pushed the record for being held in a sitting position to eight minutes.

As I was placed on the bedside, held up by physiotherapists and straps, I could do nothing. I was exhausted.

My straggly hair was rumpled and my body bruised all over. My head was bent over my chest and my arms dangled lifelessly by my sides. All my muscle control had vanished. My eyes flickered, unable to focus, and I could not see properly. I could barely breathe, I couldn't talk, and I couldn't smile.

But I had no choice other than to persevere. I had no way of refusing the physio. As with everything else, I was at the total mercy of those caring for me. After I regained some consciousness, I did my best to make eye contact with Peter during these sessions. If one of the physiotherapists asked if I wanted to continue, I blinked for yes and locked my gaze on Peter. I rarely blinked for no. Peter encouraged me to continue, safe in the knowledge that willpower and stubbornness had always worked for me; he was convinced they would carry me through this rigorous physical regimen.

My therapists were also always encouraging. They told me that with the right training, one day I might be able to walk again, even to work again. In the beginning, I reacted instinctively against the intimacy of being handled by strangers. But then I became used to it and it soon became part of who I was. The therapists knew exactly how far they could push me. What they did marked progress. I could feel it.

Not only had I lost muscle mass and lots of it, I had also completely lost any connection to my muscles through the nervous system. Most of the wiring was still there, though in some places the damage was so bad it had to regrow. If it didn't, I might never be able to lift certain parts of my body. Like a baby, I was learning to hold up my own head: tough, as the brain is ridiculously large compared to body mass. I also had what the doctors charmingly termed "foot drop" and at this early stage, there was no way of telling whether or not I would ever be able to lift my left foot. The only thing I could do was to keep trying, even if there was no reaction. The physios assured me that by continuing to push, something might happen.

Of course, no one really knew the extent of the violent pain shooting through every limb as I was hauled into a sitting position, creaking and crying, objecting to any movement after doing absolutely nothing for so long. It was as if every single joint was calcified and locked and that the slightest movement was going to break them out of their frozen positions. My therapists had learned from their training and experience how distressing this part of a patient's recovery could be, but as none of them had been where I was, and as few patients were truly able to communicate what it felt like afterward, how could they know? In those sessions I felt the physical and mental pain of being locked in, unable to share the agony and fear, while silently I screamed my head off.

Everybody was getting used to me being a mute, my communication confined to blinks or the occasional attempt to mouth words. Since my F-sound, little had happened. Every question was tailored around questions that required a yes or no answer. This took patience and skill, but as there was no other way, we all adapted. It is amazing how much you can say without words. This was our new normal.

One day while the children were with me, the nurse put the cap on the trach valve, as she often did. None of us paid any particular attention to it. Johan was dabbing ice cubes on my wounded lips to wet them and soothe the pain, Victoria was massaging my legs and Daniel, who had been telling me a story and had now finished, blew me a kiss. Suddenly, something felt different. I felt a sense of control over my mouth. I wasn't sure if it meant anything, but I was ready to give it a go. After a few carefully controlled breaths, I went for it. I didn't know if I would succeed, as my first word came out.

"Weird."

Everybody froze and looked at me. My first word in four weeks. You can fill pages detailing everything, or you can cut it all down to a single word. It was weird to talk. Weird to breathe properly. Weird not being able to move. Weird to wake up and gradually realize what had happened. Weird that so many days had just disappeared without my ever being aware they were there. Weird to look at the children and not be able to hug them.

Weird. It made my family laugh like a thousand bubbles of happiness had been released into the room.

"It's so like you to say something like that, Mum!" beamed Victoria.

That day things changed for them. A certain lightness had re-entered our lives, more familiar to our family. They started talking more around me in their normal voices, sometimes totally unrelated to me or my situation. I said very little, in fact close to nothing, but I was no longer speechless. My re-entry into the social space of exchanging meaningful sounds had been successful and was celebrated accordingly. I was still me, even if I was locked to my bed in a useless body.

Weird. It simply had to be my first word. I was unable to speak any more that day, but I felt I had summed up the situation pretty well. I was making progress. If anything, it felt weird.

A couple of days later, I was strong enough to be on the speaking cap for forty minutes. I could not yet manage an hour without my ventilator, but I was getting there.

"Tell me," I said, with great effort.

"Tell you what?" Peter asked.

"Everything," I mimed, still not strong enough to say everything I wanted to out loud.

It was always a team effort to move me, be it to wash me, put me into a sitting position, or, my newest trick, to move me into a chair. A combination of nurses, porters and therapists followed a well-tested routine. They knew each other well and chatted away as they got me ready. There were moments when the informal chatter, that special kind of laughter you get when everyone clicks, filled the room. Peter was also part of the team, familiar, ever-present, ready to give a helping hand when needed, but careful not to get in the way, enrolled in the circle of trust.

I just lay there watching them.

I knew the routine well by now. First my duvet was removed, within one minute of which uncontrollable shivers would engulf me. With most of my body fat gone, my temperature dropped dramatically. This would last the entire session. Then I was turned onto one side. I always hoped it was my right. I hated lying on the left side as my breathing didn't work properly because of the collapsed lung. I was still in pain and incredibly uncomfortable. Compared to that, the right side was bliss.

Next up was placing the transfer sheet used to lift me from the bed, making sure the straps were in the right position to pick me up. The sheet had to be tucked in behind my back and I could feel fingers trying to push it under my shoulders, arms, hips, and legs. I could hear the shuffling of busy fingers against the starched linen. Whatever position they placed me in determined my line of limited vision, defining what I could see.

This was the easy part, quick and rarely complicated, unless the nurse was new, or the porter had not attended to me before and had to get used to the sight of my hands. They always startled newcomers. Everybody tried to hide their reaction, but I noticed it every time. They couldn't take their eyes away from my dried-up, dead, black fingers. I could almost hear the questions inside their minds, and I knew for absolute certain they would ask them as soon as they were outside the room, away from my line of hearing. I was facing the ceiling. I knew every line, every corner, every tiny fault in the fittings. I could feel the group of people pulling at the transfer sheet from under my body, trying to fit it with geometric perfection for the next stage, the lifting. All the corners of the sheet were attached to a mechanical arm powerful enough to carry a very heavy human being. Picking me up was nothing. In the sheet, my arms and legs would fold as my body was held by the fabric, the only thing stopping me from dropping on the ground. I couldn't help seeing a large hole at the bottom of a sack of potatoes and imagining myself falling out.

One day as I was being lifted, the physiotherapist said, "Rikke, today you are going to try something new."

She started telling me about a "tilt table" that had been brought into my room and how today I was going to be put on it and steadily tilted until I could feel gravity in my legs and feet. Alarm spread through me.

Peter beamed at me. "This is great, honey; don't you think?" I know he was acting cheerfully in order to encourage me but, seriously, did he not see the inevitable disaster as clearly as I did?

The table was alien, terrifying, and impossible to understand. I understood the individual words, but could not make sense of their meaning when they were put together. How would you explain a traffic jam to a person who had lived her entire life in the deepest jungles of the Amazon? To everyone else in the room, it was obvious how the tilt table worked.

Usually my main concern was that while I was being lifted, someone would unintentionally tear my fingers off. It had not yet happened, but sometimes came fearfully close. At various moments in the stages of lift-off, some of my fingers were bent, pushing against the linen, and the meat and bone showed. One time my arm was caught in the sheet carrying me and excruciating pain shot through my upper body, as I thought my bone would simply snap like a twig.

At the time I was unable to make any sounds at all, but Peter caught the desperation in my eyes and alerted the staff. They lowered me down and the pain slowly dissolved and I drifted away. After that, they took greater care when lifting me. It never happened again, but the fear of something going wrong stuck with me. I was afraid, every single time I was lifted. But the idea of being tilted brought new levels of fear.

I was unable to support myself. Couldn't they see that I would collapse instantly? What if I slipped and fell on the floor? What if it all happened too quickly for them to react? What if I landed on my face and banged my head on the railings or crashed onto the floor? Could my fragile body and brain take such an impact? What if my fingers broke off in the fall and they couldn't stop the bleeding? Black, broken-off fingers on the floor, blood everywhere, and me with a cracked-open skull and my sparse remaining hair torn out. How could they do this to me? I was terrified.

I looked up—the only thing I could really do because, as with everything else, I had no say in what was done to me—and watched as the mechanical arm swung into position. The sheet was prepared, hooks were attached, straps tightened, and all the tubes and wires were dutifully taken care of. The porter pushed the button and my unresponsive body bent, head and feet levitating first, leaving my rear as the only connection between me and the safety of my bed. Then, suddenly, I was floating in the air. It took me by surprise.

I watched the distance between me and the ceiling grow. I heard the humming of the lift. I knew I was going down, but I was still horizontal. This was unusual and no attempts were made to turn me to a sitting position. My skinny buttocks served as landing gear. This was no small step for Man, no giant leap for Mankind, no Tranquillity Base. Only a miserable bag of motionless flesh and bones disembarking on a portable tilt table, whatever that was.

"Rikke, we're just about ready. You're almost in place now," came the voice of my physiotherapist, though the pounding of my heart nearly drowned her out. I was cold, my body was shaking and sweating. I wanted to go home. Home to my bed a few feet away. I heard the sound of velcro as my body was strapped to a table.

Ever so slowly the table started to tilt. It felt instantly like I was sliding down from it. Panicking, I tried to get attention with my eyes, opening and closing them, quickly, repeatedly, staring wildly into the room. No one registered my terror.

The tilt table went all the way up to an angle of fifty degrees above horizontal. I felt as if I was standing on the top of the London Eye with no railings, sure to fall at any minute. I was dizzy like crazy and ready to throw up, if only I'd had anything in my stomach. It was utterly unfair that I was too ill even to vomit.

But I didn't slide. The strap kept me in place and, seeing the tenderness in each person's eyes as they encouraged me, I knew somehow that no one would let anything bad happen to me. And if I were ever to stand on my own two feet again, I had to get used to being upright. Feeling gravity's natural pull could even be the magical kick-start my body needed in order to work again. Sometime later, woozy with the effort and emotion of the day, the significance of what I had achieved began to sink in. For a full ten minutes, I had felt gravity in my feet for the first time since I entered the ambulance in early January. I still couldn't feel my feet. But weirdly, almost prematurely addictively, I wanted more.

From then, things moved swiftly onward. That afternoon I was brought a bed-cycle, my feet attached as I lay on my back. My physiotherapist patiently started turning the pedals and my legs automatically followed, round and round in circular motions. As I was not moving on my own yet, being moved was the best alternative.

My personal trainers worked me hard, hoisting me with all their strength into an upright sitting position, never letting me go, stopping me from falling flat on my face, getting me on the tilt table and strapping my feet to the bed-cycle. I needed all the oxygen I could get and had to be kept on the ventilator during my exercises. The trach couldn't be attached to the ventilator and the speaking cap at the same time, so exercises kept me mute and focused; I was still nowhere near doing anything on my own, my body merely going along with what it was being forced to do. But it helped. Little by little I was feeling a connection to my limbs. It was wonderfully liberating.

Five days later, having progressed to a sixty-degree tilt, I was ready for the next big step, something that until recently had seemed forever out of my reach: a wheelchair, and my vehicle to getting around by myself. I had grown used to observing life from my bed. As I became more conscious, coming gradually to understand what had happened to me and the most likely outcome of my condition, I was grateful for just being alive. I comforted myself with the thought that I would see my children grow up and grow old with Peter. Any goal beyond this was not yet realistic; the idea of being able to move around in a wheelchair on my own, for example, not yet within my grasp.

The kids were there, all excited, following the details, chatting, pointing, helping, and managing to be out of the way as the preparations took place. I couldn't simply hop over from my bed. Lying flat on my back, I listened to the therapists taking me through the steps, and then looked at the world as I was floated through the air, until finally I was placed in a specially-designed chair. It was like gearing up for deep-sea exploration. Heavily loaded with portable equipment—I still couldn't go anywhere without oxygen and monitors—Johan wheeled me through the door and into the hall. It was a victorious moment for all of us, and a revelation to me—like travelling back in time, seeing the things and places that had made up the daily life of my family while I was out.

My children took me to the family room and I began to see what their life must have been like over these past weeks, all the anxious waiting, sitting there not knowing what they were waiting *for*. I saw the chairs, the couch, this small, claustrophobic room with nothing but a kettle and some teabags. I looked at the other visitors, friends and relatives in the waiting room, who may not have known what was going to happen to their loved ones. For the first time, I was able to see myself from their perspective, all the horror of standing by. I stared at the chairs where they had cuddled up, crying, fearing the worst and hoping for the best. I felt their pain.

And I realized in my heart again this was not just about me. My children needed me. I had to go even further than the wheelchair and get back on my feet.

It was another two weeks before my physiotherapist pushed the tilt table to one side. "Rikke, you are ready," she told me. "You are going to stand on your own."

She was right. I felt ready and I was ready. On the count of three, my physio on one side and Peter on the other, they lifted me and I felt my own weight on my feet, in my legs and through my body. Then I did it again.

I was standing, but it felt like flying.

It was a time of renewal. A month in, I had my first shower. First, I had to be lifted onto a special shower bed with a waterproof mattress and a hose. I couldn't raise my head to see what was going on, which I found upsetting. Next, a nurse undressed me. Being naked increased my sense of vulnerability and I was cold and afraid. But then the water hit me and it was the most wonderful feeling.

After that the shivering overtook me and I sank back into a comfortable, clean and dreamless sleep.

A new decision was made: I needed a change of scene. I was being transferred to Infectious Diseases, another highly specialized department at the university hospital.

I was not happy about that. Everything I had grown used to was about to disappear and I was terrified all over again. Intensive Care had become my unnatural home. I felt safe here and now I was anxious that I would no longer have a dedicated nurse watching over me every hour of every day and night. At Infectious Diseases, I was told, I would still have my own room but nurses had more than one patient. Was I going to be safe? What if anything happened and I needed their assistance?

Peter helped the nurses to understand my worries about not being able to call for help, so inventive solutions were tested. A button didn't work, as I'd have to be able to move my hand. A string connecting my arm to an alarm was better, but highly inefficient. It went off when it shouldn't, and I couldn't make it work when I had to. New solutions were needed, and I was still afraid. Awake, it took only a few minutes for the loneliness to creep in. I felt abandoned if I did not see or hear another person near me. The worst was to listen to somebody walking around or doing things in what sounded like somewhere next door.

What if something happened to me? What if my saturation dropped and I needed oxygen? What if my fingers got caught in something and I started to bleed? What if my heart suddenly stopped? Would they notice? Would they have time enough to react? How could I make myself known, if I needed assistance? I was miserable at the thought. The only consolation was that I was asleep most of the time. But then I woke up and it started all over again.

Contrary to my anxieties, things were going well—surprisingly well, actually. The chief physician in Infectious Diseases, who had been assigned to me on day one, as one specialist among many others, was now formally taking charge of my recovery with my transfer from one hospital department to another. I was no longer an intensive care patient, but in her care.

"Change is coming," she informed me kindly but firmly. "You need to get used to it."

Change? What did she mean? I did not want change. I wanted stability. Change was uncertainty, it was taking risks I wasn't prepared to take. But I had no say. All the major decisions in my life were taken by others and I had to tag along. I hated it and yet there was nothing I could do.

"I'm scared," I told her.

"I know. But you don't have to worry. We'll take care of you," she replied. "I'll take care of you. And we will watch you all the time. Not as closely as now. But you have nothing to fear. You'll be all right."

I didn't believe her, but it made little difference. I was moving on in my life, whether I liked it or not.

I left Intensive Care on Valentine's Day. It had served as my home for more than six weeks. Following tremendous progress over the preceding days, I had passed the last critical step to discharge. There was no trace of the bacteria in my body anymore, and the many complications arising from my infection were now under control. In other words, it was safe to move me and there was someone worse off than me who needed my room in Intensive Care.

It was always a complicated affair when I was taken anywhere inside the hospital. So far it had been only for tests and scans. Now I was really on the move, hopefully never to return—in this condition at least. All the devices and machines providing me with medicine, hydrating and feeding me had to be moved to mobile units. It took a while to prepare everything and I waited impatiently. Finally, I was released. In a state of disbelief and exaltation I was rolled out and into the unknown by a porter, a nurse, and Peter, familiar faces of nurses and doctors smiling and waving goodbye to me as I passed them.

In a film it would have been one of those sustained dramatic moments, savoring the atmosphere, a tearful send-off with people saying exactly the right thing and me replying with fluent gratitude, or at least waving silently.

Real life was different. I was a patient who was leaving, alive, not dead. They had done everything they could to get me to this moment, and now it was time to begin again and do it for the next patient who needed them. There was no time for sentiment between emergencies.

As for me, I would be only five minutes away, but it felt like moving to another country on the other side of the world.

Everything went according to plan. My new room in Infectious Diseases was kept the same as it had been in Intensive Care. Everything that had been done in my old room could be done in the new one. All the equipment I was dependent on was hooked up here; the ventilator next to my bed, the monitors measuring my heart and saturation, my feeding tube. A nurse was constantly on call, looking after me through a large window. Infectious Diseases was where patients with unidentified tropical diseases, or those attacked by drug-resistant organisms, were housed, so they were well used to dealing with very serious problems.

There was one significant change, though. Visiting restrictions changed and my mum, sister, and other family members were allowed to come more often. It was a huge relief to everyone.

"Are you comfortable?" This was always their first question, just after a quick hello. Sometimes it was my mum asking, sometimes my sister. They would adjust my pillow, my duvet, my arms or legs, anything that would add sense to their being there, providing me with comfort I wasn't getting from the nurses or therapists. Even if I was perfectly OK, I let them do it. I loved the attention, I loved them being around me. The painful loneliness that I had been suffering, locked inside myself while becoming ever more conscious and awake, started to feel a tiny bit better.

On Valentine's evening, Peter and I got a little time to ourselves, although there was very little romance about dialysis and being fed through a tube. But we were together. To me, to him, this was better than any candle-lit dinner in a fancy restaurant. We celebrated the evening, curiously happy and optimistic, among wires and monitors, the backdrop of mechanical beeps our romantic soundtrack.

After just six days at Infectious Diseases, my doctor was talking about my next move to a rehabilitation center. It felt like all too short a transition, but medically speaking, I was cured, she told me. During the past five days, I had managed to go from twelve hours off the ventilator to more than twenty hours. My wounds around my mouth were almost gone, and I was talking more and more. Sometimes I even had the strength to produce sentences with three or four words. You could hardly call it speaking, but I embraced any addition to my limited means of communication. Now, the focus of my treatment would be on physical rehabilitation—getting me to eat, to move, even to walk. Walk? I could hardly contemplate the idea. The possibility of a wheelchair had begun to sink in and felt ambitious enough. But now others had started to have higher ambitions for me.

There was still so much to do for me to be ready to move on. The breathing tube was still in my throat, as was a feeding tube that reached into my stomach. While there was still a long way to go before I'd be able to chew and swallow, there was no doubt, according to my doctor, that the air valve could go. I was not too happy about this, as it had been my safety net for so long now. When I struggled and felt under pressure, I was always allowed more oxygen. I had come to enjoy the luxury of having air pumped into my lungs when I needed it. Also, what about the hole it would leave in my throat?

"Don't worry!" said my nurse, cheerfully. "We'll tape it up!" Considering how integral to my body the valve had become, it was curious to see how easy it was to remove. It took a surgeon only a few minutes before he was standing waving it in one hand complete with trails of not-quite-healed tissue, blood and yellow pus from what he said was a typical but benign infection in the area where the plastic met the skin and flesh of my throat. He had left an open hole. Taking hold of it for a few seconds, he turned on the suction device, stuck a thin plastic tube down it, a very long way, and sucked my lungs clean from blood and slime.

There was a lot. It hurt like crazy and I couldn't breathe for the full minute he took to finish. To him it was routine, like vacuuming the car before handing the keys back to the owner. I wanted to kick him and stick the tube down his throat, so he could feel the pain and misery himself, but then he was off. Besides, I could barely move my leg, so kicking was out of the question.

The nurse cut the tape and closed up the hole.

I could feel the tape blow up like a small balloon when I blew air through my mouth. The patch was changed regularly and as there was no sign of infection, I was assured that eventually the hole would close.

Now more than anything, I wanted to be with my children, to talk to them, answer them, play with them, walk with them, eat with them, read to them.

To be their mother again. My dreams soared.

EIGHT

Walking

In Intensive Care and Infectious Diseases, they had tended me, cared for me, brought me back to life—and now that I was no longer in danger, their job was done. It was time for me to move on to the next stage of my recovery. After forty-nine days at the university hospital, I was transferred to one of the best rehabilitation centers in the country.

My emotions were mixed. I knew this meant I was going in the right direction, but it also felt as if I were being cast out to fend for myself, a bit like leaving home to go to college. I knew there would be people to help me, but I also knew that I would have to be more independent.

I was given a room in the Early Neuro-Rehabilitation Clinic—a section for patients with very little cognitive ability and movement. My room was small and white, unwelcoming and horribly unfamiliar. Everything felt wrong about it. Peter tried to cheer me up and arranged my photos so that I could see them from my bed. But it didn't help that much. And it turned out I was still utterly dependent on others, except in a strange, new environment with new people and strict new rules and routines. It was so difficult adjusting and I woke each morning with a growing sense of dread.

Ever since being admitted to hospital, my kidneys had not been working properly. When the first drops of urine had appeared in my catheter bag, this had been a major turning point and a reason for optimism, as it meant my kidneys had started working again. Not very well, though, and my doctors in Intensive Care thought it might never come to more than this. But ever so little was better than nothing and even if I were to be on lifelong dialysis, it would be assisted by my own body, and as such was a sign that I had begun to contribute to keeping myself alive. This had been an important step forward, the foundation of self-respect. I was proud, simply because this was something I could do on my own.

At the rehabilitation center I was still stuck with my catheter bag, transparent and yellow. It had faded a little as a symbol of triumphant survival and was beginning to become a bit of a problem, a reminder of what I couldn't do and of my utter dependence upon others.

One morning, as I lay in my bed, two nurses were talking across me.

"Where should I put the jar?" said one of the nurses.

"Just put it by the door," replied the other.

They were deciding where to put the urine they had emptied from my bag. My eyes followed their movements. Still unable to talk very much or move more than a fraction, I lay there following a conversation as if I were not present.

"Be careful not to spill it," the second nurse continued.

"Do you remember when I accidentally kicked a jar and that urine went all over the place?" the other nurse replied, laughing.

"Oh yeah, I do! The tube went whirling around the room and we were all soaked in urine. Don't do that again!"

"It was pretty disgusting," said the first nurse, a mixture of amusement and disdain in her voice. They started laughing as they turned away from me. I felt so vulnerable and humiliated, unable to maintain even the minimum of dignity. Peter wasn't present, so I had nobody to fight for me. I began to cry.

But my crying was silent. The sound of crying, a high-pitched wail or a low hollow moan, is a statement. It says: I am here, this is my pain, this is my grief. In my solitary prison, I could not even do that to make people feel or see my pain. Despite all my progress, I couldn't make people see how much I needed to be recognized and respected as a person, not another faceless, brain-damaged patient. I had a face, and it was streaked with dried-up silent tears.

Peter had been by my side every day since the New Year. Now it was March. He had to go back to work at the university.

Working in one city, visiting me in a different city and taking care of the children in yet another city was a logistical challenge. Now, he came to see me on his way to or from work, but only for an hour or two before he had to leave to make it in time for a meeting or pick up Daniel. The first of those endless days, when he wasn't there every hour, I cried.

"It's a sure sign of depression," said my new doctor. "No doubt about it. It's perfectly normal, given your circumstances. I see this all the time." She straightened her back. Job done. She was already walking away, on to the next patient, leaving me in my white room, engulfed by loneliness. I *was* sad. But I was not depressed.

My left eye had been watering for a few days, and like a tiny biological tap, it just wouldn't stop. I could not lift my arm to dry or wipe it. I simply had to put up with it. But I knew that her diagnosis of depression was wrong and through the intricate means of communication Peter and I had developed—subtle signs in how I looked at him, blinking, lip-reading, using the spelling board that was driving both of us crazy and throwing in a few words every once in a while—I told him to tell the doctor that I was not depressed. In fact, I was over the moon with all the progress I was making, ready to make more. There was simply something wrong with my eye.

But she didn't listen to Peter. She relied on the information she gained from reading the charts and whatever she could glean from the patients themselves. As this was almost always very little—there are limits to what immobile, brain-damaged patients can communicate effectively, let alone expansively—she was used to relying on her own experience and expertise. She ignored Peter as he conveyed key information about how I had been treated at the university hospital, despite the fact he had spent two months meticulously going through all my reports, analyzing the test results and tracking down the latest research. I had asked him to be my voice and now I felt my doctor wasn't listening to me. Peter was there to help and to act on my behalf, but in her domain, there could be only one person in charge. This was not his business.

I had no way of summoning my limited abilities to tell her how I felt. She saw on me a frozen grimace of pain, my facial muscles locked in an expression I wasn't feeling. My body had no language and I had no proper voice. I could whisper a few words, but even then, you really had to know me in order to understand what I was saying. She had no patience for that. Throwing a quick standard diagnosis at me—brain-damaged and depressed—she could tick the box and get on with her job.

But this was too important. I had to tell the doctor that I was happy to take the next step, to feel and gain a little more control of my body. I felt so full of power and initiative. This particular rehabilitation center, I had been told, was my golden ticket to regain a life beyond hospital walls. She had to know I was not sinking into a black hole, and I was ready to prove myself. All that was happening here was that there was something wrong with my eye, and if she would only take a look at it, she would see it was no impediment to progress. Peter understood me perfectly. He told her that both he and I thought there was something wrong with my eye, that I wasn't depressed. But she held her ground, insisted it was depression and that it would be treated.

Three days later, less than a week after arriving at the rehabilitation center, all I could think of was how to escape. I was going insane with the overwhelming desire to get out of there. OK, I couldn't move much, which was a bit of a challenge. But there had to be a way for me to get hold of enough bed sheets, tie them together, throw them out of the window and climb down from the third floor to the street. Then I would have to find a way to hitch a ride back to the university hospital. If I had any chance of surviving this, I had to leave. Unlike my previous stream of delirium, I was totally in control of these thoughts, a sure sign of progress, if not a reflection of reality.

I told Peter, "I want to go back to the hospital." A difficult sentence to say, and it took me some time.

"There's a different doctor on duty today," he said. "Let's try and talk to her before we make any plans."

Fortunately, this doctor was a good listener. Through a combination of verbal and non-verbal communication, we told her everything. How the nurses paid no attention to my cognitive abilities and how her colleague had ignored our concerns. We told her how my tears were a response to feeling so humiliated and we were pretty sure that humiliation was not the same as depression. And finally, somebody took me seriously, believing that there was something wrong with my left eye.

"Thank you," she said. "I'm grateful for your honesty. We rarely have patients in this unit who are able to communicate how they feel. I am so sorry we have made you feel this way and that your concerns were not taken seriously. We need to get you moved to the Sensory-Motor Clinic, where you'll be able to continue on your journey of recovery."

And she was as good as her word. Two hours later, I was told that a room would be ready for me the next day. I cried again. But this time from relief. Somebody had heard me.

And I got a patch to cover my damaged left eye.

Settling in my new surroundings, I started to believe in progress. That first week had been absolute hell. But now, at the Sensory-Motor Clinic, I was finding my bearings. It was a new world, a land of opportunities. People were moving around in wheelchairs on their own, they were sitting in the common room—talking, eating, listening to a particularly gifted nurse as she entertained us on the piano. And then there was Michael.

I never learned all the details of Michael's illness, but that didn't matter to me—all I knew was that he was the coolest guy around. We had been in the same place, locked in a body that couldn't move. I had my bacteria, he had his virus, and we had both gone down all the way, until there was very little hope and almost no prospect of recovery. But now Michael could walk. The first time I saw him he was standing tall, legs kinked, a body wobbling like overcooked linguine. But he was on his feet. I was impressed, intrigued, and wanted to tease every secret out of him.

"I'll ask him to come over," a nurse said. She told me how Michael had been sitting like me, unable to move a muscle. How he had been in a coma and through months of rehabilitation. Standing in the open door to my room, he introduced himself and we started talking. Well, that was a bit of an exaggeration. He talked. I wheezed.

"How?" I rattled. Thinking this might not make sense, I elaborated with a faint "What?"

"You simply need to believe that you can walk. Never give up," he said and then outlined the regime of exercise and physio he had undertaken, telling me that any progress, however small, was significant and could be built on. He beamed with confidence and was clearly trying to inspire a novice. I *was* inspired. I *wasn't* going to give up. I *would* be walking.

At that moment this was totally out of reach, of course. At my best I could sit in my wheelchair, but only for brief moments at a time, barely able to hold my own head. In fact, I had a head-rest that went around my neck, covering my ears, making it possible for me to look ahead, but not to my side.

Michael made me see that looking ahead was important in more ways than one.

Every patient here had suffered some kind of brain damage. And it seemed to be indiscriminate in its scope—children, young, old, strokes, accidents, injuries and a range of abilities. Some patients were able to walk and talk, others could only sit and stare—shells of their former selves.

I came to see that survival here was all about hope, the most important fuel to our brain-damaged engines. Without it, getting—or being taken—out of bed for another identical day of confusion and failure might have been futile, for both the patients and their relatives. If you woke up with the hope that today was the day you were going to pour yourself a cup of tea, or make a conscious decision to get to the breakfast room and eat cereal with your new friends, then you were on the road to some form of recovery, even if you were never going to be able to make yourself tea again or get yourself down to breakfast.

But hope was also the heaviest burden and one that many patients couldn't carry for themselves. My doctor told me that she often made a contract with her patients to carry it for them, to keep it alive. When I wavered, I had Peter and my children, my parents and sister, my in-laws, friends, and colleagues to help me keep going. But it didn't take away the fact that every day was miserable. I was beginning to lose faith, lose sight of ever returning home again. I hated my room, hated the bare walls, the clinical cabinets, the medical equipment, the many outlets to run the machines, the lift in the ceiling, my metal bed and hospital clothes. I hated everything about being at the hospital, about losing my old life and being unable to see what the future would bring. I tried to hide it, but failed. Peter noticed and started thinking about what he could do to cheer me up.

One day, waking up after an afternoon of strenuous exercise, I sensed something had changed. It always took me a while to get my bearings, to get the strength to open my eyes and persuade myself for another round of whatever was planned for me. At first, I didn't see it. Somehow the light had changed, or the color of the room, but I couldn't quite put my finger on it. And then I saw it. Everywhere on the walls and the cabinets were large prints of me and my family, enjoying our adventures around the world.

There we were hiking the mountains, showering in a waterfall, walking along the coast, sitting by a quiet lake enjoying the sunset, exploring a city, going through a

Cambridge college, everyone happy and all of us together. I was overwhelmed by the physical presence of our memories of happier times; they flowed through me and gave me an empowering feeling of resourcefulness.

I was back on track, despite the hardship, and ready to push through. I had a visual of my target and decided to take everything to the next level.

Peter was sitting in a chair in my room.

"Hey, honey. I thought you needed something extra," he said with a quiet smile. "Do you like it?"

I loved it.

"I've also bought you some new clothes. Track suits, some cool T-shirts, that sort of thing. I figured that's what you need right now. Let's get you out of these hospital rags and into something more suitable, your own stuff. It's about time you stop being ill and start being yourself."

I couldn't agree more. He pulled his chair over to my bed, and we went through every single image, every memory. That night I had the best sleep of the year so far.

Having the pictures around my room and being able to share our memories was very reassuring. It meant my brain was still in some ways intact. It was the thought of being brain-damaged that I found hardest to bear. I could see the signs in people around me—drooling or unable to control themselves, stopped in their tracks. But that wasn't me. I fashioned myself as a survivor. And yet here I was.

You could only be in this unit if you were brain-damaged and being in this unit was my only way to recovery, possibly even my ultimate salvation.

I knew that I had been saved from serious brain damage. Blood clots had formed deep in the very base of my brain—too many for the doctors to count—and in the front right side was a swelling of blood and fluids that had stopped, by a hair's breadth, exactly at the right time before pushing against the barrier dividing the brain in two. Had it not stopped there, I would have been beyond recovery, a vegetable forever at the mercy of others.

Despite this, there was still not a doctor in sight who could say confidently what the long-term consequences of the clots and the swelling would mean for me. Clinically, I was brain-damaged. In the months to come, I learned that this could mean a whole lot of different things.

Lying awake, listening to the nocturnal sounds of machines and murmurings, I composed my list of physical desires: to feel the ground under my feet, to have the muscles in my legs flex, to feel the weight of the rest of my body, to put one foot in front of the other. I tried to block out the fact that I still couldn't even place my feet on the floor, that they would not do the things I wanted them to. They just fell down, like two tiny sandbags tumbling out of a wheelbarrow. It was as if they had lost all connection to me.

There I was: a patch over my eye; hair falling out; dry, black, crooked witch fingers; hollow cheeks and a bony body. But Michael had done it. He had found his feet and made that connection between them and walking. In thinking about Michael, in thinking about standing on my feet, swaying, unstable, ready to collapse any moment, I could touch the sense of freedom that he had gained. I stopped seeing myself in a wheelchair. I saw myself walking like Michael.

"This is what I want," I told myself, over and over. "This is my future."

But I was still utterly dependent upon others. I could only move very little. Breathing was a constant challenge. I communicated in brief, hoarse gasps with the hole in my throat covered. I could not eat and was still receiving nourishment through my veins. I was wearing hospital clothes, despite Peter's best efforts. My bed hummed constantly from the generator that blew warm air through the special mattress that prevented bedsores. When my temperature dropped, I was warmed with an electric, air-filled duvet. When my temperature rose, layers were removed and I was cooled by chilled air. My body was unable to maintain a constant temperature, and infections, immediate and aggressive, were an unremitting threat.

Now the focus was on occupational therapy, on finding a way to do everyday tasks, like being able to hold an object, take a bite of a sandwich, lean back in a chair, or use the remote control. I was beginning to think that some fine day, I might be able to do all that. Perhaps I would even be able to put on my own underwear, the new ones that Peter had bought, and be free of the baggy, coarse hospital knickers I'd been wearing for the past two months.

I hadn't had a thing to eat through my mouth since the first of January. All my nutrition was now fed to me intravenously as I was losing weight, down to just forty-five kilos. The intravenous food made me nauseous, and I was frequently, sporadically sick throughout the day and night. Having lost all use of my muscles, I was unable to swallow. There was simply no connection between them and my brain, as if all the wires had been cut.

To that end, a tiny camera was inserted through my mouth into my throat, and a blue staining liquid was then poured in. I hated it. The nurses could see my distress and they tried to reassure me. "It's nothing to fear," said one. "I've tried it." But what did she know? She was healthy. She had control of her bodily functions. She could pretend to try. But she was in no danger of choking. When the liquid hit my throat, I felt as though I was drowning.

What does it take to swallow? More than twenty muscles, even for a tiny bite. Now, in order to eat, I would have to train my throat muscles to work.

It all came as a complete surprise to me. No matter how hard I tried, I could not control anything going on in my throat. The blue liquid flowed down, making me retch and cough. I was choking, my swallowing reflex gone.

I loved sucking on ice cubes. A nice nurse saw that. "You're thirsty? Right?"

I was, and I longed for a proper drink of water, just the sense of it, the satisfaction of quenching a thirst that had lasted for months.

"Let me get you some water. This will make you feel better."

It did make me feel better, but at the same time it made me worse. Inadvertently, she poured water straight into my lungs. As I couldn't control my breathing, I was unable to cough and thus the water stayed in my lungs, gradually filling them up rather than my stomach. I was still so out of touch with my own body, I didn't register that something wasn't right. A fever began to build. My malfunctioning immune system could not fight off another infection on its own as bacteria grew exponentially, thriving under perfect conditions. The humid, closed environment that constituted my lungs was a perfect biological breeding ground for pneumonia.

Luckily, I was monitored so carefully that anything even a bit out of the ordinary was clocked. I was quickly put back on antibiotics, but my body suffered from the setback and my training was put on hold. Small steps in the wrong direction could make me go downhill fast. One out of four mechanically ventilated patients get hospital-acquired pneumonia and around 10 percent of them die.

Even off the ventilator, I was at great risk. The blue liquid test was a crude but effective measure of how much of what I was drinking went into my stomach and how much went into my lungs. At first my throat didn't discriminate, but little by little, with enforced perseverance, I got better at it. Still almost without any muscle control, I was beginning to sense the minute difference when something went down the wrong tube and within a couple of weeks, my reflexes woke up.

I knew I would never get out of there if I could not eat for myself. I had no body fat left. I was a skeleton with some poorly functioning intestines and skin holding it all together. I had to gain weight and come off the intravenous drip. I was constantly fighting nausea caused by the complex pattern of being locked in with physical damage to my brain and months of lacking proper digestion. With a great deal of patience and training, I was beginning to swallow soft or watery substances. "Super" ice creams—the fattiest, most disgusting food ever invented—and cucumber (one of the few things I found would relieve my nausea) were introduced to my diet. I hated the ice cream more than anything I had ever eaten, and the cucumber had no calorific content. It didn't work. I did not put on any weight at the rehabilitation center.

It was a tough regime. Days were packed with exercises or tests. A typical day would include some activity in the morning, a symbolic "lunch" with a therapist and exercises in the afternoon.

I was utterly exhausted by the late afternoon when the kids and Peter visited. Eating was difficult, both physically and mentally. Chewing and swallowing was still uncomfortable. I didn't want to eat with the other patients. I had no appetite and my fingers were disgusting. Or rather: I was afraid others would find my fingers disgusting and then not be able to eat. My fellow patients ate in the common room, but I stayed in my room during every meal. In between activities, nurses, doctors and therapists would come into my room several times a day to talk about progress, plans and targets.

My favorite time with the staff was when they came in with no assigned task, only to hear how I was, or talk about normal, everyday stuff. Not my medication, not my fingers, not my diet. Just asking what I used to do, what I dreamt of doing, and commenting on things happening in the world. All my strength went into physical and occupational therapy. I didn't have a drop of energy for the outside world, but I liked to hear about it nevertheless, a bit like playing on the kitchen floor when I was a child and my parents listened to the radio.

I had to get used to being at the hospital for long periods on my own. Some days, when the loneliness became too unbearable, I had a nurse call my mum. She was always available and would make the two-hour drive to see me any time of day, stay for a bit, then turn around and go back home, usually before Peter and the children came in the evening. She tried to keep herself together when she saw me. Sometimes she managed better than others. I could see during every single visit how much everything pained her and yet how much better it made her feel that she was doing at least something for me. Still, it did not stop the agonizing internal loneliness I was feeling day in and day out.

Aside from my daily regime of therapy, there were also other specialists who came to see me, checking my fingers, my diet, my well-being. One morning, a wound specialist knocked on my door.

The hole in my throat had closed up, and I had now become better at speaking—though my conversation was hardly flowing.

"Come," I said, as she entered my room.

The wound specialist had come to take care of my fingers while they were in the process of breaking off, to clean the wounds in order to avoid new infections. But today, spotting my messed-up feet, she exclaimed, "Rikke! What's going on here? Have you seen your feet! We need to do something about this!"

She was right. My feet were in a terrible state, the skin ruined by medication and lack of movement. I was used to decisions about my care being made by others, but this time, I silently agreed.

She went out of the room, returning a few moments later with two plastic bags and a large bottle of sparkling water.

She poured the water into the plastic bags and placed one foot in each, tightening them with rubber bands around my ankles. After thirty minutes of soaking, she gently peeled the leathery skin off my feet like ripe fruit. I was horrified and delighted at the same time. When she'd finished, they felt soft, like baby feet.

As I got stronger and more independent at the rehab center, my world started to expand. I was spending more and more time in my wheelchair and no longer had to be lifted into it. My hard, physical work was paying off and ultimately I was strong enough, with some help, to slide myself from the bed into my chair and I was getting pretty good at it. Still attached to tubes and wires, I was beginning to enjoy a higher degree of freedom.

Daniel loved pushing me around in the wheelchair and, when I wasn't in it, he would commandeer it himself, scooting around my room, turning tricks on its wheels. If he felt adventurous, he would speed down the halls, skillfully avoiding any oncoming nurses and patients. I loved seeing how fearless he was, and wished I could act like that again someday. The very thought of driving through the open door, out into the daylight, feeling the wind against my face, accelerating down the wheelchair ramp and coming to a standstill at the roadside made my heart beat a little faster. I would be in perfect control of my driving machine. When Victoria and Daniel came after school, they would often wheel me down to the games room, and I sat and watched while they played board games and table tennis, catching up on everyday things with Peter. This was the normality I had craved for months.

My therapists were taking me farther and farther from the safe confines of my bed. Eventually, we made it down to the gym. This was no ordinary gym, with quiet areas for occupational therapy, lots of highly specialized equipment for severely disabled people and a small pool. At the very back there was a tiny room with weights, the only thing familiar to me. That room was like looking at the moon. I could see it, but going there seemed impossible. Peter was by my side as we were introduced to the equipment, and the physios outlined the training program that I could now embark on. As one of them wheeled me around, she stopped at a set of railings, a few feet apart with a short track between them.

"One day, Rikke, you will walk along here," she said. They had already learned—the doctors, nurses and therapists—that I thrived on challenges. When they presented me with options that would push my limits, I wanted to have a go. If anyone suggested there was something I couldn't do, I wanted to prove them wrong. I looked at the track, about five meters long. She knew I would not let this one pass. She was cleverly baiting me.

If I didn't take her concealed invitation to give it a try, no harm was done. On the other hand, if I went for it and didn't fall flat on my face, this might very well be the next step in my recovery. Of course, I couldn't resist the challenge. I looked at the track and the bars as the habitual feeling rose inside me. I didn't want to wait. I was ready.

"How about now?" I asked.

"Sure," she said, glancing at Peter. He smiled and nodded silently.

She wheeled me to one end of the bar and asked Peter to stand at the other end.

"OK," she said. "I'm going to remove the chair, but don't worry, I'll be holding you. You won't fall."

She lifted me up and held me as I dragged my feet, putting one foot in front of the other. I walked all the way toward Peter. In this moment of victory, I would like to have smiled, waved or at least said something, but I was focused on having another go. My legs were already cramping and my arms were shaking, but I wanted this, I needed this. Peter and my therapist helped me turn around and once again I saw nothing but the track in front of me.

I walked the stretch of the bar twice that day. I was ecstatic and so exhausted that I knew I would sleep the moment my head hit the pillow. I had done it. I had walked.

It was a momentous achievement for me. To Peter it was also extremely special. He had watched all our children take their first steps and now he had also watched me relearn how to walk. There was still a long way to go, but I was getting there.

This was on the sixteenth of March. Exactly two and a half months since I had last taken a step.

One of the nurses mentioned that a hairdresser who came regularly to the center could see me. It sounded like a good idea. I quickly realized that it wasn't.

As she wheeled in her cart, she shot one quick glance at me while reaching for her tools.

"No one will notice the bald spots when I'm done," she said. "We should take away what is left of all your long stuff and cut it short. Short hair will suit your face You'll look much younger."

Was she crazy? Anybody who took one look at me would think I was eighty years old, even though I had not yet turned forty.

My hair was falling out, I was wearing a black eye patch, my fingers were drying up, I was bone-thin, and I couldn't smile, not even a little. I had no control over my facial muscles, and I looked old and angry, miserable and resentful, with my lips turning downward in what looked like a hideous dismissal of everything around me. This was not me. This was not how I felt. I looked at myself in the mirror. I was ugly. How could the world see me as anything else?

She did her best, but it made little difference. There was no magic makeover.

I had heard some of the other patients talking about home visits. From where I was lying, home might as well have been on another planet, though I did allow myself to imagine opening the front door to our house and walking through to the kitchen, the heart of the house, with its huge table where we ate and talked our way through meals; sitting in the study, where the children did their homework and we talked about the books we read; and finally, going into our bedroom and getting into bed with my own warm, fluffy duvet covering me. I longed for it.

So, when the doctor suggested it one day, I couldn't believe that elements of this fantasy might come true.

"Yes!" I beamed. "I want to go home."

"You're ready for a short visit," she said. "A nurse and a physiotherapist will go with you, but it can only be for a couple of hours."

She could have said anything beyond "you're ready." All I wanted to know was when.

Three days later, I was strapped into my wheelchair, having been pushed into the specially adapted van that was bringing me from the rehabilitation center to home, excited beyond belief. As we drove, I looked out of the window, wanting to take in every little change of environment: the snow on the pavements, the icy trees on the roadside, the gathering storm. People were walking along the street shopping, talking, normal everyday things now so very unreal to me. The light was too painful, and I got only a glimpse of the real world. I was so easily exhausted. I closed my eyes and fell asleep, well protected, feeling safe. I had never visited my own home before. It was a strange, almost exotic feeling, bathing me in a lightheaded happiness.

Turning onto our road, a quarter of a mile from our house, the van got stuck in the snow. We were trapped. If the van couldn't drive on, there was no chance of me getting into my house. The snow was too deep for my wheelchair and it was far too dangerous to leave me out in a freezing temperature for more than a few minutes, even with all my blankets and warmest clothes. I was just sitting there, strapped down and locked inside the van, unable to do anything, so close to home. After all this effort I was not going to make it.

But there was no need to worry. Peter and Johan came running toward us and with the help of a passing neighbor, the nurse and the physiotherapist, they dug the snow from around the wheels and pushed the van free. Eventually we were able to continue the final stage of our journey. There was no way we could make it all the way onto our drive, but Peter and Johan had dug a path in the snow for me. My nurse tightened the blanket around me and Peter pushed me in my wheelchair out of the van.

How I'd longed for this moment. How many times I had imagined my home, room by room, the light, the warmth, the memories, the familiar scent of our house. All that is home. Peter and the children had made the house comfortable for me: a portable ramp got me through the door and things had been moved out of the way for ease of access. I would like to be able to say that Peter lifted me from the wheelchair into our winged armchair—my special comfy chair—and that I sat there for a couple of hours basking in the warmth of my home, the children close around me, talking, laughing, cuddling me, while I retook possession of our house. But I was nowhere near doing that.

The fact is that I was utterly overwhelmed and exhausted from travelling. All I wanted to do was to lie in my bed and feel the comfort of our mattress under my bony body, hear the rustle of the duvet cover and breathe in Peter's smell. And so it was that I pretty much slept through my first visit home. I had to be woken up. We had to get back before the storm picked up and darkness fell. There was no room for risk.

The next time home was easier. The snow had gone and I got to stay a bit longer. Two weeks later, Peter was even allowed to take me home on his own. He had made a beautiful selection of my favorite foods: small portions of homemade hummus, lentil paste, bread right out of the oven, avocado, fresh mango, grapes and strawberries, cranberries and nuts. It looked delicious, but I had no appetite. I was still fighting constant nausea and only managed to eat half a strawberry.

It didn't matter. I was home. This time, with the children at school, I was alone with my love, just like in the old days. We had the house to ourselves. I was all bubbly inside. Feeling adventurous, even slightly reckless, I immediately fell asleep in a soft cloud of sheets.

Now I could walk a bit *and* I was sitting up out of my wheelchair for longer and longer. My rehab room was fitted with a winged armchair, balancing independence and support. But I was still unable to pass urine myself. It was time to get my bladder working again. My catheter was taken out and an elaborate process began. Every third or fourth hour, nurses came in to empty my bladder. A bedpan was put under my buttocks and I was told to pee. In the beginning I couldn't really feel anything. After what seemed like an eternity, a handheld scanner was used to determine if there was any residual urine. Remaining urine could cause additional infections and, in the end, kidney failure. If the scanner detected any remaining urine, a catheter was put in to empty the bladder completely.

Every time I hoped it would be the last. It never was, and for more than two weeks I had to endure the bedpan-scanner-catheter regime until, finally, one day I had emptied my bladder by myself three times in a row. I was full of joy, especially as it had an added value. I could now wear my own underwear. Having my own panties on made me feel ecstatic. They were so tiny compared to the hospital knickers, so delicate, so perfect.

Spring was on its way, flowers in bloom. Victoria's birthday was coming up. We were used to being together on birthday mornings, and it meant a huge amount to all of us. I told my doctor about Victoria's birthday and she asked me if I wanted to spend the night at home. I had less need for the feeding tube, which had opened up a host of new possibilities in terms of training, eating, and, now sensationally, a sleepover at home.

On the day before Victoria's birthday, Peter took me home. He had prepared a meal for me and tried to hide how nervous he was. I still had no appetite, feeling constantly nauseous, every single bite a physical nightmare.

"I'll be in trouble if you don't eat," Peter said.

I tried, but failed. There was nothing I could do. It was physically and emotionally impossible. I knew in the long run that this had to change, too, if I ever wanted to leave the hospital. But I wasn't ready for it yet.

Sleeping at home was independence; familiarity and devotion. I still needed help with everything, but it gave me an element of control. I was beginning to notice how my family was behaving. I could tell if Victoria had experienced a bad day in school. I could sense if Daniel would rather be playing with his dinosaurs than talking to me. I could see how exited Johan was to be able to hang out with his dad watching old movies into the night. And I noticed that Peter had a lot on his mind. He talked to me about some of it, but tried to hide the rest. I knew he didn't want to worry me, but I could read him like a book. We talked about our life post-hospital, or rather, we settled into our routine of Peter talking, asking questions, and me lending a nod or a brief comment every now and again, mostly just a word or two.

He planned to put in a permanent ramp for my wheelchair and make a series of other adjustments around the house. Unsure if I was ever going to be able to return to work, he was contemplating how we would manage on his income alone. We would probably have to sell the house and move to a smaller place. We didn't delve too deeply, but we were both increasingly preoccupied about how different our lives would be.

In the morning we celebrated Victoria's birthday. As I watched her open the presents I didn't buy her, I thought, next year, when she turns sixteen, I will be buying her present, I will bake the cake, we will plan her day together. I will be her mother once again.

As Daniel put on his coat to go to school, he looked up at me. "Mum," he said, "do you think you could walk me in to school?"

Absolutely not, I thought. It was a crazy idea, but I didn't have the heart to tell him.

I looked at Peter. He nodded and we silently agreed to give it a try.

"I'd love to," I said, thinking how impossible it would be. I tried to control my nerves. I wanted to be strong for him. Peter helped me into the car and we drove Victoria and Daniel to school. When we arrived, we walked the twenty yards through the playground into the primary school, Daniel gently holding my hand. He smiled up at me, his eyes shining, and I thought, I've done it. I have done what he asked me. But it wasn't quite over.

"You coming up to my classroom?" he asked.

His classroom was up a flight of stairs. I had climbed steps in the gym, but this was a different scale of challenge. I looked at the stairs. I could just as well have been staring at one of the most dangerous climbs in the world.

"I don't think so," I said. "If I make it up, I'll never make it down."

"I'll help you, Mummy," he said. "We'll do it together. Take my hand."

And I did. Suddenly he was no longer my eight-year-old son. He was a strong and independent young boy taking care of his mother. Helping me to put one foot in front of the other, comforting me every time the pain and cramps became too much to bear. Stopping on every step, and after what felt like an eternity but was probably only five minutes later, we reached the summit. It was one of the most moving moments of my life. To watch my son become my hero, my guardian.

At the top, after climbing twenty steps, I was shaking, sweating, thinking of my hospital bed. I was completely wasted, while Daniel was beaming the most wonderful toothy smile, proud beyond belief.

"You made it, Mum," he said. "You made it!"

NINE

Cutting

My fingers, blackened and withered, served as a constant, painful reminder of what was to come. The more active I became, the more I could do, the more they were in the way. I was afraid they would break off accidentally when I was wheeled down the hall or moving from my bed to my chair, or that one of my hands would get stuck under me and my fingers would rip off one by one.

I had been told from the beginning that the idea was to wait until they broke off naturally, but as this became more imminent, I started dreading it more and more. It wasn't that I didn't know how to prepare mentally for losing my fingers; my fear went far deeper than that. I was utterly terrified by not knowing how to live a life without them. I looked at my impossible hands, useless black claws, and I cried with my entire body, as if every single molecule was unhappy. It happened every time I looked down, every time I thought of my fingers, every time they were in the way, when they got caught in the bed sheets, in my clothes, in the wires that still connected my body to the bag of white stuff I was consuming through my veins. Every single time, I felt the pain of losing them forever, for good, and there was nothing I could do about it.

My hands were suffering from gangrene, very similar to what happens when mountaineers get serious frostbite. You can get gangrene from a whole range of different things: injuries, diabetes, long-term smoking and infections, but the result is the same. Blood circulation is shut off and your cells die. Another name for gangrene is necrosis: death, the stage of dying. A dead cell cannot be brought back to life. When it dies, it is gone. When many cells die quickly, the body cannot replace them with new cells and that particular part of your body is closed down.

This is what happened to me. As soon as my body had shut down my skin got dark, cold, dry and hard, but when I woke from my coma I had already stopped feeling anything and had lost all sensation. I could still see parts of my body, but it was as if they didn't belong to me anymore. Something that used to be me was dying, drying up and mummifying right in front of me.

Traditionally, gangrene has been dealt with by cutting off dead limbs before it spreads to the rest of the body. But as the orthopedic surgeon had patiently told me several times over, while my fuzzy brain tried to take in his words, the newly perceived view was that you could keep more of what was left of your body if you let the dead bits fall off by themselves. It also helped the healing process once they were gone, and it helped another problem I would inevitably face.

As an amputee, you have to live with an invisible experience. A part of your body is gone, but it still hurts, madly and maddeningly. These are called phantom pains. They are real and they are really painful. They feel like they are coming from body parts that are no longer there, but they sit in your brain and your spinal cord, not in your lost limbs. If your leg is cut off, you will continue to feel the pain in a missing foot. This is normal when a healthy body is dismembered. It is difficult to treat, and it seems so unfair that something you have lost forever will carry on giving you pain. But if the body is left to process a dead limb gradually, rather than simply cutting it off quickly, nerves will die a natural death and you are left with less pain in the parts that are gone. If you suddenly cut off the nerves in the human body, you mess up the rest of the system. If you let them part a little at a time, they will come to terms with it and leave you in peace.

By this point, I had no sensation whatsoever in my hands. It was unbearable. I wanted them off, I wanted them on. I couldn't bear to look at them and I couldn't stop looking at them.

Broadly translated: I had to sit and watch my fingers wither and die until they fell off.

They were ripe. Like milk teeth still hanging in there on a tiny fleshy wire. Ready to fall out, or, in this case, to fall off. I could see the bone and the flesh. Black. Red. White. This also meant my hands were packed with open wounds, perfect conditions for bacterial growth that had to be fought off constantly with antibiotics. Worried I would not be strong enough to fight off any further infection, my surgeon decided that it was too risky to wait any longer. They would have to go a bit earlier than planned.

They were in the way. My previously untroublesome fingers that had served me so well. My little finger on the right hand was a particular troublemaker: curled up inside the palm, it effectively blocked any movement in my hand. It became painfully obvious. I would be better off without my fingers.

So much of me was defined in my hands.

Age four: I plunged them into soft clay and a perfect replica of my hands emerged. This was something we all did in preschool—I did it and, growing up in a different part of the country, so did Peter, and so did our children. Like thousands of parents up and down the country, my mother had put my cast in our living room, a reminder that my hands had once been so small and perfect. Now, I asked my mother if I could have the cast. I needed to have my hands, if only as a hardened memory to hang on my wall. But it was long gone.

Age eleven: We were playing tag in the school gym, chasing each other, laughing and shrieking with delight. I ran toward the toilets with a girl at my heels, chasing me. I was fast, could dodge even the most determined chaser, but she was getting closer. Shooting out of the gym, I slammed the heavy door. I can still hear the sound of my finger getting caught in that door, my scream as the tip was cut almost straight off. I looked at the piece dangling from my index finger, only attached by a tiny string of skin. My teacher acted swiftly, and I was sent to the emergency room, the bit of my finger in tow. Fortunately, it wasn't too late for the doctor to stitch it back together, eventually leaving nothing but a tiny scar. I treasured that scar; it was one of my defining features. No one noticed it, but to me it was special. Through the years it served as a reminder of what I had almost lost.

Age twenty-three: Drawing and painting were a huge part of my life. Before completing my degree in science, I decided to take a sabbatical to explore that side of me. I enrolled in art school and enjoyed every single moment, even considering applying to the Danish Academy of Art. In the end, I chose science and went back to university, but a part of me never left art behind.

Age thirty: I was seven months pregnant with Daniel, and the four of us had joined in a game of rounders at the school fair. I was fielding. As one of the batters sent a hard ball flying, I reacted instinctively, my body flying through the air, precisely as I had taught it to do during my years of football training. As I prepared for the perfect landing, I realized too late that my center of gravity had changed. Everyone froze as I landed straight on my pregnant belly. But before anyone could react or rush over, I was on my feet, holding the ball over my head. I may have floated through the air like a slow-moving blimp, but my hands did not betray me. The point was ours.

I have always been a fighter, never willing to give up. Even now, almost four months into my hospital stay, I hadn't lost my spirit. I liked being in control and little by little I was retaining a bit of it in the gym, in my physio sessions, by breathing, eating, moving and walking. I was getting better. Every week was marked by rapid physical and mental progress. I was moving my body around. It wasn't elegant and it wasn't quick, but it worked and I was able to do more and more all the time. I was constantly breaking barriers and fighting to achieve the next goal. But faced with the loss of my fingers, I was drained. I was losing far more than my fingers. I was losing control and I was fearful of what was waiting for me.

But beyond even that was my terror of letting go. The surgery to remove my fingers required a general anesthetic, and I was petrified that I was going to lose my mind—again. Being in a coma had changed me. I was now sufficiently recovered to know how lucky I had been to wake up the first time. How likely was it that I should have that luck again? What if something went wrong? Would I have to start all over again? Had everything for the past couple of months been in vain, fighting for survival and another chance in life?

When an iceberg melts, it makes huge ponds of fresh water in the ocean. Layers of different kinds of fluids sometimes create a rare physical phenomenon leading to liquid zones. This is what happens when freshwater ponds suddenly appear in lots of saltwater. A boat can sail into it with everything working perfectly, engine running, propeller churning. But suddenly it will stop and no matter how much power is used, the boat will not move. The surface remains calm. For the crew there is nothing to see and nothing to do. This phenomenon is called dead water.

This was me. Inner turmoil, all engines roaring at full speed, but on the outside no expression. Composed. Placid. Dead water.

I couldn't bear the thought that there was even a minute chance I might wake up after surgery without any memory. Or that I would not come out of surgery, slipping back into a coma. Or worse. And more than anything, I didn't want to put my family through any more pain. All this raced through my head. I cried, screamed, shouted, raged, cursed, tore the curtains down, threw all the things I could get hold of at the door, smashed the mirrors. All on the inside.

It was one day around this time that Peter brought me the news about the bombing of the Boston Marathon. I couldn't take it in. We used to live in Boston, when we were both working at Harvard. We have many happy family memories of weekends exploring the city. We tried not to miss a thing. The marathon was special, the world's oldest annual marathon and a celebration of what can be achieved when you push the limits. It had taken place every year since 1897 on Patriot's Day, the third Monday in April. Had we been in Boston on the fifteenth of April 2013, we would most likely have been standing there in the crowd. Knowing my family, we would probably have pushed toward the finish line. Some of us might even have been taking part. We went back to Scandinavia, but we kept Boston in our hearts.

A beautiful day turned into a bloody mess of panic, pain, lost lives, and lost limbs perpetrated by two twisted minds. I felt the pain and hurt, the agony of the destruction. Three innocent people were killed and more than two hundred and sixty others were injured. A young boy, almost the same age as Daniel, lost his life. All that potential, all those dreams and aspirations, lost in a single arbitrary moment. I cried and I could not stop, tears running down my face. I cried for the victims, for the families, for the city. I cried for all of us, for all the things we lost that day. And I cried for those people who had lost parts of their bodies and out of nowhere had to adjust to a new life.

I thought of how many lives had just changed. I knew I was lucky. The survivors were lucky. Like many of them, I would soon be an amputee as well. It was all so unfair and none of this should have happened.

I closed my eyes and wept again.

The first time I tried to hold a pencil to paper at the rehabilitation center, I cried. Nothing worked. I had no control. My black fingers were in the way, and even a toddler's scribbled lines looked better than what I was able to produce. I hated it. I hated everything about what had happened and the consequences I faced. I hated not being able to keep my ability to visualize every thought on paper as I was used to.

But it was so much more than that. It was some of my fondest childhood memories, the precious moments with Daniel and my everyday escape. Daniel's drawings and Peter's prints of our family adventures were decorating the walls of my room. One of the photographs showed me in the Angeles National Forest, sitting under a tree next to a stream, drawing. A happy moment. No one could tell me, in losing my fingers, if I would ever be able to draw again and I simply didn't know how I would deal with that loss. I did not know if I could. And I didn't know what a life without drawing would mean.

But I had another test to face first.

"Hi, Rikke!" The neuropsychologist knocked on my door. She was here to pick me up for cognitive tests recommended by the chief physician.

I was skeptical, had no idea what was expected from me. A lot of thoughts were flying through my head. What would she find? What would the consequences be? What would they write in my medical chart? Could it be something that would affect my chances of holding on to my job? I told myself that I had to shine, that I needed to be utterly convincing. I told myself this, but I wasn't sure how to do it.

Sitting in front of this woman, accustomed to being professionally nice, I couldn't escape the thought that my fingers were letting me down. My own hands were so pathetically useless and while I could speak fairly well now, with my left eye only half open and the serious trouble I had controlling my facial muscles, I could barely see the test sheets put on the table in front of me. But I was not going to let this defeat me and so I gathered myself up to take it on. I had to be alert and ready.

She was friendly and asked if I was ready. I nodded. At first the tests were straightforward and I did well. "What's the next number in this row?"

"Which geometrical shape is missing here?"

"What is twelve plus eighteen, minus four, times eight, plus thirty-two?"

"Start with one hundred and keep subtracting the number seven."

"What's the odd one out when looking at these cards?"

"I'm going to tell you a story; please tell me what you remember and preferably in the right order."

On the first of three scheduled tests, she kept going for almost two hours, firing questions at me with no break or time for reflection. This was repeated three days later, but with new questions, and again ten days after that. I was exhausted each time, but in a good way. I knew I had done well. I was confident that there was absolutely nothing wrong with my cognitive skills in terms of intelligence, memory, language, planning, or problem solving. I was playing on home turf. Working through the tests, I had been pleased by her tiny signs of surprise when I got the really hard questions right.

After she had analyzed the third round of tests, she told me, "You were above average in most of the tests. You did really well. Did you enjoy doing them?"

I did, so I smiled.

"But there were minor problems that we have to consider," she continued.

I didn't like the sound of that.

"Some of your tests covering executive skills, such as the ability to think of new ideas, might not be as good as they used to be. You might find creative thinking difficult as a result of what has happened to you."

I couldn't believe it. Was she serious? Had we been in the same room during the tests? I tried to compose myself and took a deep breath, carefully phrasing the sentence in my head before asking her, "What are your reasons for reaching that conclusion? Which tests support this?"

I was shocked, and I couldn't hide my surprise. She was startled by my lack of immediate acceptance of her verdict. After a brief, awkward pause, she explained that the main reason for her concluding that my creative thinking had been damaged was how I performed in the verbal fluency test for words beginning with the letter S. In this test, I'd had to say as many words as possible that began with the letter S, in one minute. I'd managed ten words, not bad for a person suffering brain damage. But it was below the average of a normal person and compared to my other results, it stood out as poor.

I was very upset. I could not believe anyone would base an important conclusion on such a poor data set. Thinking as a scientist, everything about that was just wrong. She was sitting right opposite me presenting her verdict, daring to take away my creativity. In all of my professional and scientific life, this had been what defined me. But still, this was what went into my medical chart: *The trauma to Rikke's brain has caused a loss of creativity and ability to problem solve.*

I was furious. I felt beaten down, casually brushed aside as the person I used to be, the person I was fighting so hard every day to become again. I couldn't believe it. The doctors were taking away my fingers, and now she said I was losing my creativity.

I was determined not to let this happen. I was going to prove her wrong. Of course, she had no idea of the effect on me. To her, taking tests with patients, analyzing the data, and providing results was what she did. To me, however, it was personal. The interpretation of the test results was about who I was and who I could still be. In a curious sense, she did me a favor and helped me to focus my mental powers much more clearly. I was going to leave with my head held high, and I was going to live a creative life. I needed to believe that, if I was ever going to get out of there and pick up my life again.

And then it was time. I had been transported back to the university hospital and the surgeon told me in great detail how he was going to remove my fingers, while holding up a pair of pliers for demonstration purposes. The pliers took me by surprise. I had envisaged a tiny surgical saw and other precision instruments, him working delicately on each finger one after the other, carefully sewing up what was left with surgical thread. My imagination was somewhat off track. I wanted to know everything and yet part of me wanted to know nothing at all. But my curiosity got the better of me. Would each finger break off easily or would some be stubborn, not wanting to part from my hands? How would he sew up what was left? I became obsessed with the details and wanted to be there as my fingers came off. I wanted to bear witness.

"Are you ready?" the surgeon asked.

No, I thought, and forced a smile as I heard my own voice saying, "Yes, of course."

All procedures were followed and everything went according to plan. The anesthesiologist put me under as the surgeon suited up. Nine of my fingers had surgery and were partially removed. I slept soundly and never felt a thing.

When I woke up, I looked down. Two white, bandaged boxing gloves, looking like small white cantaloupes.

Other than that, there was nothing to see, and I could not help feeling slightly disappointed. I had been thinking about this for so long and had been so worried. I had cried, I had talked endlessly to Peter about it and I had been very, very quiet, keeping most of my thoughts to myself, never letting my guard down and allowing the doctors and nurses to see what I really felt. I didn't want them to think I was weak or scared. But I had been scared, of course, scared of everything: the procedure, waking up without my fingers, my reaction, and how I was supposed to get on in my life using my new hands.

Gazing at my gauze spheres, now with signs of blood seeping out, I still didn't feel anything. They were numb. But that didn't last long. Soon the pain started and it became real. They were really gone, my beautiful, wonderful fingers, my dexterous friends. Now it was over, irreparably over, and there was no turning back. The magnitude of what I had been through finally sank in. My life would never be the same as it was before I had become ill. Never. I was now physically changed in a way that could not be reversed. The pain from this was different. Something else inside me broke, never to heal.

After a few days, the surgeon began to unroll the bandages, gently freeing my hands more and more. I thought time would stop. I expected horror, grief, tears and shouting about the unfairness of everything at anyone who came near me. But that didn't happen. More than anything I was curious to see my new hands, what the stitches looked like, and how much was left.

This was the first day in my new life. I was eager to discover what my new hands could do. I wanted to try them out. I wanted to get out of the hospital, start over, get on with everything–and go home.

TEN

Leaving

I watched the specialist nurse clean my wounds, making sure everything was all right, carefully checking for infections. I watched the doctors examine my hands and all the time I watched the remnants of my fingers. I don't know what I had imagined, but this was different. At the very least, I thought the wounds would have been delicately closed up with tiny stitches, so small you could barely see them. This was not the case. Flesh, blood, and bone were visible. Strings were sticking out and you could see the knots. How they would ever heal was beyond me.

I followed every tiny change, watching my fingers as they healed. Every day the scab changed, little by little. The threads became more visible and the wounds more tender and swollen, a sign of healing. And when thin bandages were placed over the tip of each finger, my hands started to look surprisingly normal. The bandages were changed each day and the wounds were improving.

When you cut fingers off with pliers, your skin and flesh do not contract at the same rate, leaving your skin sitting kind of tube-like around the flesh and bone. These edges were steadily pulling inward as new skin began to form. It was a relief that the dead parts were no longer in the way and as I got used to my tiny hands, I found myself more adept, my movements quicker. As an exercise, I was handed a pillbox with seven compartments, one for each day of the week. My task was to use my new hands to carefully divide my weekly doses of medicines into each compartment, and, day by day, I found myself able to do it.

It was not all going right. My left eye was still a mess. Doctors had tried to find out what was wrong with it. I had even been back to the university hospital on a day trip for specialists to have a look at it. I could not see anything but a blur when I closed my right eye, and I was told that it might never be any better. My cornea was damaged, making me practically blind, but it still reacted with a painful sensitivity to light. I couldn't see and yet, ironically, I was blinded by the light and had to protect my eye. The eye patch had become increasingly uncomfortable and reminded me constantly of my illness. I longed to escape that, so instead, I had taken to wearing sunglasses at all hours. By now, I was able to put them on and take them off by myself, and if I had my way, I kept them on.

I was also having trouble with my left foot. It bent inward and got in the way, making me stumble, causing me problems as I made progress walking. A cast was fitted to keep the entire lower part of my leg in place, and I had to wear it as much as possible—even sleep with it. I had to endure the uncomfortable itching, the numbness it triggered and the distress of not being able to put it on myself. I joked about how pirate-like I was. I had the eye patch, the severed hand in need of a hook and the "wooden leg." I only needed a parrot on my shoulder to complete the picture. If I was ever going to walk properly, I had to give the cast a chance.

Around the same time, a clear fluid had started to run from my nose. It was incredibly annoying and came at all hours of the day and night. I didn't have a cold, so the fluid needed to be tested. It was a painstaking job and not a very nice one for the staff. All the fluid from my nose had to be collected. Every time I had an itch or felt something watery in or below my nose, I had to call a nurse. They would come running with a vial to collect the fluid. If I had to blow my nose, all content would have to be collected too—*all* the content.

Collecting my nasal secretions was quite a show, embarrassing and exhausting. The first batch turned to gel while being transported to the lab and couldn't be used, so it had to be done all over again. The doctors had a suspicion that the fluid might be coming from my brain or spine, which would be critical. The brain is a delicate organ, packed in a hard shell of bone and floating in a liquid to protect it from bumps and injuries to the head. If the brain leaked, it would lose one of the two main protective agents. To everyone's great relief, the tests revealed that it was neither brain nor spinal fluid. In order to figure out what it was, and where it was coming from, it was necessary to have my entire skull scanned.

The images revealed a cavity in my sinuses that was a potential risk for bacterial growth, hidden like a microbiological terror cell. Surgery was needed in order to prevent the constant and detrimental risk of further infection.

Once again, I was scared. Not only would this mean a general anesthetic, going completely under, but this was the first time I was to have surgery inside my head. Just as I was regaining control of my mind and body, I would have to let go once again and leave both in the hands of others. I was terrified of the darkness and depth of a coma, and I felt helpless and marooned all over again.

Despite the fact I had recovered from surgery before, I was unable to get over the possibility that this time I would not wake up, that in saying goodbye to Peter and the children, I would be doing so for the last time. But there was nothing I could do. I had made a lot of progress, enough to realize what a fragile state I was still in and that things could go downhill fast. This was a necessary procedure for me to get well. It was not about my recovery anymore; it was about my future life and trying to prevent everything from happening again.

I kept my worries to myself and braved a smile. "No problem! I'm ready! Let's do this!"

As it happened, this was only a minor surgical procedure, a standard operation that could be done at any hospital. The staff acted accordingly. In my mind, however, it was always about life and death. I recovered quickly, feeling no different after the operation, and within a few days my runny nose stopped. As it had already been established that I had neither a leaking brain nor spinal fluid seeping through to unwanted spaces, the doctors relaxed and the focus was once again on getting me on my feet and working on the biggest remaining issue: weaning me off my white bag of liquid protein that I still took through my veins.

I was still nauseous all the time, constantly fighting a strong feeling of vomiting, day and night. It prevented me from sleeping well. The nurses tried everything to make it go away, all sorts of medication, but nothing worked. Finally, they were left with nothing but the hypothesis that it was my body rejecting the intravenous food, so I was promptly taken off it and left on my own to gain weight.

And so there was no way around it anymore. I could not get away with chewing a few grams of cucumber or sucking on half a teaspoon of ultra-fatty ice cream. I had to start eating properly— the last real breakthrough I needed to be on my way home. I was still eating alone, but I began to eat a little more and then a little more, and finally I was able to manage without my white bag. As a result, I lost even more weight, but I was eating just enough to satisfy my doctor that I was on the right track. After a couple of weeks, my nausea began to subside.

I was feeling better. Every week I was breaking records, now being able to walk down the hall—not on my own yet, but I was putting one foot in front of the other. Most of the time was still spent in bed. I continued to sleep a lot, but I now enjoyed sitting in the armchair in my room. I could see the window from there. Spring was coming. I wanted to go out, but although my range had increased,

I was not yet able to leave on my own. My family took me around the hospital in my wheelchair when they visited. We had settled into a new routine.

Peter was again busy at work and keeping everything afloat at home with the kids. He still visited me every day, the kids took turns most weekdays after school, and on weekends they all came. I knew how important it was they returned to a kind of normal life, spent time with their friends and did all the usual things for their ages. They were playing, reading; they watched films and played video games. I wanted to join them and continued to push myself in the gym, taking every new challenge that was thrown at me. I was beginning to get used to my new hands. They took a long time to heal and they were completely different from what I knew. But they were not bad. Not at all bad.

At the rehabilitation center I started getting more visitors. Friends and colleagues stopped by for a quick hello. With a few exceptions they were all shocked to see me, a fraction of a second's hesitation as they entered and first laid eyes on me. They tried to hide it, didn't mention anything, but I noticed everything, every time. At least the children quickly got used to it and acted perfectly normally around me. My mum cried each time she saw my hands. Trying not to make her feel worse, I felt I couldn't really tell her that she had to get over it. I had to get over it myself. I had to get over everything. I had no choice. I was stuck with my new hands and everything that went along with them.

I was going home more frequently and each time was a small victory. But there is something inherently wrong about visiting your own home. You should never have to do that: You should simply go home. And I had been away for so long that even as I went back more often, I couldn't help feeling removed from things. Shattered as they were, my family had managed to carry on with their lives and there was so much I had not been a part of. Daniel had been a troll in his drama class production; Johan and Peter had bought new bikes; they had been to the movies, gone to concerts, been at parties. I had missed out on it all, and so, I resolved, it was about time that I took part again, full time.

It was a daunting prospect. I had been totally dependent on others to look after me, to decide what I needed and provide it. The thought of going back home in such an altered state, making decisions again and determining my own day, as far as I could—to participate in normal everyday life, even with help—was both scary and exhilarating.

Quite apart from the emotional adjustments we would all have to make, there were practical considerations. Would I need someone at home caring for me while everyone was out at work or school? Would I need help getting dressed or using the toilet? If I was alone in the day, who would help me to take my medication? I took twenty-nine pills every day, ten in the morning, six at lunch, six at dinner, and seven at night. In my current state, that was a meal in itself. If I wanted to go home, I had to do this on my own. There would be no doctors and no nurses next door to tell me what to do and when to do it. I had to step up and take responsibility. There would be no safety net.

One morning, I walked Daniel in to school. I was due to go back to the rehabilitation center, having spent the night at home. Daniel helped me from the car, guided me through the doors and held my hand as I climbed the stairs.

When we got to his classroom, he asked me to come in and as he was taking off his coat, his teacher came over.

"Rikke," she said. "Is there any chance that you could stay around this morning and answer a few questions that the children have about what has happened to you? Daniel has been so good at explaining things to his classmates, so eloquent and patient and as a result they have so many questions."

Daniel beamed. He touched my hand gently.

And before I knew it and without any preparation, I was standing in front of twenty-five children trying my best to answer all the difficult questions, all the ones adults are far too polite to ask. Eight-year-olds are brutally honest. They say what they think and before long they were firing questions at me, as if we were in a verbal shooting range.

"Is it true you slept for two weeks?"

"Why do you look so old?" (*Did I?*)

"How did you learn how to walk?"

"If you were dead, are you a zombie now?"

"Your hair looks funny and you are very thin."

"Are bacteria really that dangerous?"

"Why do you stay at the hospital?"

"Don't you want to go home?"

"Will your fingers ever grow back?'

And as I looked around at their attentive, interested faces, I realized that I could answer as freely as I wanted. It was such a relief to be able to talk openly about all these things.

"No," I said, smiling at them, "my fingers will never grow back. They were cut off, because my blood had stopped flowing in them and then they died. Just like when you pick a flower from the garden. It will survive for a bit, but it won't get all the water and stuff it needs, so it will wither. It was a bit like that. Except my fingers withered before they were cut off.

"I look old because I have been very, very ill.

"I was in a coma for two weeks. It is very much like sleeping, but it just goes on and on and it doesn't even make a difference if you set the alarm. It takes a very long time to wake up. Some people in a coma never wake up. I did."

I explained, "When you lie in bed for so long, all your muscles get weak and can't support your own body anymore and then you have to spend a lot of time training to do all the things none of us think about, but just do. Like walking. Jumping. And sitting down in a chair in front of the computer without anyone helping.

"And yes, it is true, my heart stopped. But sometimes when that happens and you have the right equipment, you can get the heart started again. I was lucky. Someone was there, and they knew what to do. I am just as much alive now as all of you."

Daniel, who had been standing by my side, squeezed my arm. The teacher thanked me, but the children were fascinated, unable to let me go without asking another battery of questions.

"Because of all the medicine I had to take," I continued, "I lost almost all of my hair. It just fell out when the nurses combed it. I still can eat only teeny tiny bits of food. I get most of my food from a bag of white liquid. I have a small valve attached to my arm and it comes straight into my veins. That's why I look so funny with strange hair and a bony body. It was bacteria that did all of this to me. Some bacteria are good. They help you digest all the food you eat. And some are bad. Like this one. It can give you a cold or a fever. Or, if you are really unlucky, it can make you very, very sick.

"I'm still too weak to manage for too long outside the hospital, but I can visit you and I can visit my family in our home. I work hard every day at the hospital on my physical training and I am getting stronger and stronger. I want nothing more than to go home—for good."

Daniel was listening intently. When one girl asked how the bacteria looked, Daniel jumped in, "It's so small, you can only see it with a microscope!" He was on top of it. He didn't miss a beat, and not for a single moment had he hesitated or flinched, not even when the really tough questions were asked. My little man, doing so well in front of his classmates.

"Thank you so much for sharing your story with the children," the teacher said. I walked out with a feeling almost of elation. I had stood there, Daniel at my side, and talked about everything. No longer afraid of who I was or who I had become. I sensed happiness at last.

I needed to prove to myself that I would have a fighting chance of at least some degree of independence. And so, back at the rehabilitation center, I hatched an ambitious plan. I kept it a secret from my family and worked it all out in my mind before involving anyone else. I was quite good at being with my own thoughts by then. I thought out every last detail, the mental gymnastics tiring and complex, for my brain was still not firing on all cylinders. First, my plan involved getting some money. This was tricky and it took a few goes before I felt I could ask Peter about it without arousing any suspicion.

There were various things I could pay for at the hospital. By having some money and not having to ask Peter for it each time, I could make an argument about keeping my dignity, and he would see this as a step toward my independence and full recovery. Then I had to calculate the absolute shortest distance to the place I needed to go, and then work out if I could make it. Walking was the only option I was allowing myself. Being taken there in the disability van was not part of my equation, with all the lack of independence it implied.

I also needed the right equipment to execute my plan, but as all I required was pretty basic, I didn't think this would be a problem. It was only when I had figured it all out that I allowed myself to think about an accomplice, someone who could keep quiet, help me through all the stages and, most importantly, not dismiss my idea out of hand.

I knew exactly who: my occupational therapist. She would understand and approve of this challenge. But I would need to think deviously. If I could somehow get her to think up the idea, work through the details and worry about whether it was really possible, and then let her slowly convince me until I gave in, that might succeed. It was a cunning ruse. But in the end, I didn't need any of my guile. I could sense an open goal. So I told her everything from the beginning of my plan to the end. She thought it a brilliant idea and all my therapists soon went along with it. They saw it as a great sign of mental and physical recovery. I saw it as a victory.

I was entering the real world again. I was going shopping.

The shop was only a quarter of a mile away, but it may as well have been in Timbuktu. I had to get dressed to go outside, put on shoes and walk along the pavement. This was a different world from anything I had experienced the entire year. My physio had brought a tiny backpack for me to carry my groceries in. There were other people on the street; cars and bicycles sped along so fast, and it all felt loud and overwhelming.

Walking to the store was the hardest thing I had done in months. But with my physio by my side, I slowly and carefully kept putting one foot in front of the other. It took more than half an hour to get there. The responsibility of the project was mine. It was up to me and no one else. I was so enjoying myself. I had to walk in and find the things I needed, put them in the basket and walk to the register. It needed my full concentration. Despite the change of scene, I hardly noticed my new surroundings. I just kept my focus on not falling and on getting the goods.

"You did it! That's incredible," my physio said.

But I still had to get back to the hospital, and then the real work would begin. Time was of the essence.

In the late afternoon, Peter and the children came to see me. I suggested we have tea in the kitchen. Some of the other patients were sitting at the other end of the table. They had waited patiently for this moment.

"Could you get something from the fridge for me?" I asked Peter.

The other patients had heard about my voyage to the supermarket and had been monitoring the entire operation from the sidelines. Now they followed Peter's every move as he opened the fridge door.

"That," I said, pointing to the big round cake in the middle of the bottom shelf. "I made it for you."

I beamed. Peter took a couple of steps back.

"You made it? For me? But how?" Euphoric with pride and happy beyond measure, I took Peter's reaction in as he tried to make sense of it all.

"Look what your wife has made for you. You must be so happy," said one of the patients.

It was Peter's birthday, and I had decided he should have a cake. One made by me.

"Mum, you made a cake. You're amazing!" Johan and Victoria were as proud as their dad and couldn't stop smiling, while Daniel was jumping up and down with excitement. It was a victorious moment—not only for me but for all of us. We had been through so much pain and grief together; now it was time to share some happiness. Peter cut the cake.

The piece of cake on my plate remained untouched. I smiled. My eyes were closed. I wanted to taste it, but I could not even open my mouth, let alone lift a fork that far. There was nothing left in me. I had to lie down. Sleep was coming up on me fast, a matter of minutes now.

The children were chatting away; Peter was talking to Victoria. "Will you excuse me?" I said. They barely noticed. And as I started to move, I was overcome by a sense of wonder. I had set myself a goal, thought up a workable plan, got dressed, put on shoes, walked to the supermarket, bought ingredients, and made a cake from scratch. Every step had been intricate and tough going, totally disproportionate to the end result, but what I loved was seeing my family eat the cake, chatting to whoever they were sitting next to, barely noticing that I was nodding off; it all felt normal, as if it was merely something I could do, like I used to. I loved it for its ordinariness, for not being anything special. An everyday thing.

"I'm sorry, you'll have to excuse me," I tried again. It was the shortest birthday party ever. But it was the best. They all helped me to my room, tucked me in and left quietly. I fell asleep within a heartbeat. Hours later when I woke up, I felt the happiest I had been in a very long time.

Change was in the air. After the cake, people started getting practical around me. The focus shifted toward getting me home permanently. I felt different, too. I looked at the newcomers, some in wheelchairs, some in beds, unable to move or talk. I was feeling better, stronger, more optimistic. I was growing out of this place and it was time to move on. It felt reminiscent of the time when I realized—and my parents did, too—that I had outgrown home and was ready to move out and become independent. It had been a powerful feeling back then and was even more so now.

Peter and I talked to a social worker. This was a first, but now I was part of the "system" and she was here to help me make the transition from long-term hospital patient to being on my own, living at home. There were all sorts of things to consider. There were medical bills to take care of, we had to organize help at home and start thinking about finances. Was I entitled to any benefits? Could Peter support us on his salary if not? Could we keep the house? Could I keep my job? Would I ever be able to work again? How should I react if I felt ill? Who would make the tests and collect all the blood samples? So many things to worry about. So many clear and present dangers. And yet, I couldn't be more excited.

And then one day, it was time. The chief physician was smiling in a way I had not seen before.

"Rikke," she said, "you're ready. Somebody else needs your spot here far more than you. It's time for us to let you go."

I was going home. I knew from the chief physician that most people at the rehabilitation center were afraid of going home. Afraid of what they might not be able to handle. Of what they had to face on their own.

Not me. I couldn't wait. I spent all day getting ready to leave. Nurses and therapists helped me pack and made sure I was informed about every little detail I needed in order to move on.

I would not lose contact altogether. I was sent home, but not yet formally discharged. I was given a phone number to call if I needed assistance, but I would be half an hour's drive away and would rely on someone else to take me if I needed attention. I was overwhelmed by the level of information, feeling I was forgetting something critical. In reality, everything followed protocol and was under control.

At half past four in the afternoon, Peter walked in and then we were heading home—for good. I thought about the first few days at the rehabilitation center when I was so miserable that the only thing I could think of was how to get back to the safe confines of the ICU. I thought about how much things had changed, how much I had changed. I was stronger now. The next step felt perfectly natural. I was like a bear coming out after a long winter's hibernation. I had said goodbye to patients and staff during the day, and now to the nurses on the late shift. It was an emotional day, but also wonderfully practical. To me my life had changed, but to everyone else at the rehabilitation center, it was just another day and there was work to do. There were hugs, a few tears and then Peter took my hand. "Are you ready?" he said.

"Yes." I smiled. "I am."

And as I walked out of there, smiling, holding Peter's hand, I promised myself that this was it. I would never go back. I had never been happier to be going somewhere else. In the car, Peter played a song for me from the new album by one of my all-time favorite bands, EELS. Since my student days I had felt a strong connection to Mark Oliver Everett's music and lyrics, the sincerity and authenticity of both the light and the darker sides of human existence that only comes from personal experience.

The first song was "The Turnaround," about a person who'd had enough of being written off and decided to head out to a better life. I closed my eyes and let it all sink in; everything that had happened since the violent bacterial attack, the coma, being locked in, desperately trying to communicate that I was there, blinking, using the spelling board, learning even the most basic bodily functions all over again and now this, driving home with Peter. I was feeling wonderful, glorious.

The fifth of June is a special day in Denmark, celebrated as Constitution Day. But to me it will always be Independence Day—the day I returned to life, to my home and my family. I was finally free and in charge of my body and my life again. As we drove up our street, the flags were out.

As we parked in our driveway, the children came running out. Johan opened the car door and they all helped me out and into the house, bubbling with joy.

"Mum! Mum!" they cried as they huddled around me like happy penguins. There was so much to say, but we needed no words to tell each other what we felt.

I wanted to take it all in, to keep every single thing as a precious memory, to see, touch, feel and listen to everything and everyone. I wanted to walk around the house, go into the garden, to eat and drink; I wanted to sit in my favorite armchair with our cat, California, on my lap.

But all I could do was to go straight to bed. This was where it had all begun on the first of January. But now, after more than five months away, it was again a happy place.

A couple of days after getting home, I sat down at our kitchen table and wrote an email to all the friends and family who had supported me over the past months. It was something I had wanted to do for a long time, but I could not until now. It took me hours and I had to think about every sentence. I had to write with tender fingers and was really only able to use the thumb on my left hand. I had lots of flowers and cards around me; I was wearing my own clothes, while the children were somewhere else in the house and Peter cooked our dinner. I looked out of the window at our lush, green garden. The sun was shining, and I couldn't help smiling. It all went into my letter.

"After 153 days, I'm home!" I wrote. "I have used every word, every thought, every drop of love and friendship from you to fight this." It was difficult for me to express how much it all helped me to get back on my feet. But I told them I had been through hell and it wasn't pretty, and that all their cards, letters, and emails from near and far made me see the light at the end of the tunnel. Everything helped me when the loneliness became almost too unbearable, when my strength was lacking and the constant struggle seemed pointless.

I explained that we were supposed to be in Berlin over the summer. Everything had been planned carefully last autumn. Peter had been offered a visiting professorship and at the time we were looking forward to a new family adventure. But as a result of all we had been through, we changed the plans and were now spending our first full summer in Denmark in seven years. Looking back, our life had been a series of changes, moves, new towns, new houses, new jobs and new schools. But everything had been planned meticulously. Nothing had been left to chance. We had done everything together and because we wanted to. We had taken the opportunities as they came along, but we were always thinking long-term of what would be best for our family, for the kids and for our careers. We had been in charge of our lives. Now life was in charge and we had to change accordingly. That was new to us.

I finished my letter. Dinner was almost ready; time to call the kids to set the table. But perhaps there was still time to go and sit in my favorite spot in the garden under the warm evening sun.

I didn't have to ask anyone's permission. I didn't have to tell a nurse where I was going.

I could just go.

ELEVEN

Living

I was weak, I had to gain weight and I still needed lots of physiotherapy and medication. It was going to be a very long time before I could ride a bike, go for a run, drive my car, or get back to work. But I could get started, all in my own time. I could go with my family to a strawberry field and eat as many berries as I could manage; I could sit in the shadow of a tree and read a book; I could sleep in my own bed, next to Peter, and enjoy a Sunday brunch with the family.

But most days I took life as an adventure. I was overwhelmingly grateful. I noticed everything. I enjoyed the sunlight flickering in the fur of our sleeping cat. I listened to our children talking about what happened during lunch break at school. I watched Peter sleep. I was grateful for all the little things I had taken for granted, all the things that make up most of our lives.

Now I stopped, looked, listened, took in the smells: the flowers in our garden, newly baked bread, my children's hair. I loved it; I couldn't get enough. I wanted to get the most out of everything. I didn't want to miss out on anything. There was a new intensity to living and everything it entailed. I had received a gift: the gift of appreciation, of not wasting all the everyday adventures that are right in front of us. The gift of making every single day count.

At the beginning, everything was new. Hospital had been so different and even though I had learned to live in hospitals as if they were my home, they weren't. Now everything at home was challenging and although Peter and the children helped all the time with even the tiniest things, I felt as if I was fighting like never before. Everything exhausted me. Walking down the hall to go to the bathroom, managing my way to the conservatory, or checking the mailbox by the end of our drive—it wore me out and I was constantly looking for places to rest.

One of the things I remember best from the first day was sitting down, eyes closed, and just listening to the life of the house, noises I had never noticed before: what it sounds like when sneakers are kicked off in the hall, tea is being poured, or the difference between a cat coming and going through a cat flap. I learned to navigate the sound universe of my home and knew exactly where everyone was and what they were doing, at least as well as if I had my eyes open.

I had a nurse come once a day, but apart from that we were on our own. She checked my bandages and medication, and asked me quickly how I was. She was sweet, but on a tight schedule and out of the door before I could answer her question. It was such a huge difference from the hospital, where I had staff around me all the time and I could always call for assistance. I had never had to wait more than a minute. Now I had to wait for Peter or one of the children, or I had to do whatever I wanted or needed myself. Peter was helping with most things, but I really wanted to do everything myself. It helped. I got better and stronger every day. I even started to eat more, although I still had no appetite. But I knew I had to get on with it if I wanted to get my strength back. Friends and family came around and I started to hear news from work. I enjoyed the visits, but tired easily and was poor entertainment.

I wanted company, but also had to accept that everybody else was leading their own lives, had to go to work and do their things. A lot of our family and many of our friends lived far away and couldn't just come over for a cup of tea. I could write only a few lines a day, but loved hearing from everyone, to feel connected.

When I was lying in my own bed, enjoying the wonderful feeling of a completely normal bed without strings, wires and alarms and thinking about how far I had come, I realized that even though I was permanently suffering from loneliness at the hospital, I had never been alone. There was always someone next door.

Being alone was new.

So I learned to let go. The children had to go to school in the morning and Peter had to go to work. At first, he didn't like leaving me on my own, and I wasn't too happy about it either. What if something happened to me; what if I fell and couldn't get up or was unable to reach for the phone? And what if I suddenly got ill again, like on New Year's Day, but this time no one was around to save me? But none of that happened and we both knew it had to be done. I had to start taking care of myself.

I had always worked and never spent extended periods of time at home on my own. It was a new and very strange experience. I was too weak to do anything around the house and had to leave all the practical everyday stuff to the rest of the family. California and I had a lot of time on our hands and we did all sorts of things in our tiny world, exploring all the good places for a snooze and finding exactly the right spots in the house and the garden. Together, we read one book after the other and all the time I was getting stronger.

Every other day I was picked up to continue my exercise and physical therapy program in town, at the local rehab center. I joined a group of people who had suffered strokes and were also trying to get their bodies to follow orders again. There wasn't anyone who had experienced exactly what I had, but all of them had their own stories to tell. Many shared them, some were silent. Most of those recovering from strokes were over seventy. I hung out with the "younger crowd," a couple of guys in their fifties, and I enjoyed their company. We set ourselves targets and could beat the "oldies" most days by at least two push-ups and eight minutes on the bike. Piece of cake.

I knew I had been changed physically by the bacterial infection and all the implications that followed, but the scale of the consequences were not immediately obvious. My shock as I struggled to do the laundry, to make tea, to take a short walk, or sometimes simply trying to stay awake was profound. It would take a long while, years perhaps, for me to get back into the shape I was before the coma—and maybe I would never reach the same level of fitness, or have the same kind of stamina as I'd once had.

I might be on lifelong medication, always having to carry antibiotics with me to be on the safe side. When I finally came off my medication, if I did, Peter would have to learn how to inject a life-saving shot of antibiotics in my leg, just in case. I would never regrow a spleen, and although a vaccination against pneumococcal infections provided me with very good protection, it didn't match the natural biological defense I lacked. I had to take certain measures and I would have to learn to adapt.

And then, of course, I had to adjust so many daily routines. The most obvious ones were: buttoning my shirt, fastening zippers, opening jars, and picking up coins at the register. Sometimes I asked Peter to take me to a shop, to make me feel I was a normal human being doing normal things. I liked getting out, but buying things was also annoying, not only for me, but for the customers waiting in line behind me, unaware of why it was taking me so long to check out. I was often embarrassed, and I thought how unfair it was that I wasn't given any extra space and time, and that people should understand right off the bat and be more patient.

Then there were the awkward things, like not being able to get things out of packets, or not being able to pick up popcorn as the bucket got passed down the family line when we were watching films; shaking hands with missing fingers, or forgetting about my hands when pointing something out, only realizing too late that I had nothing to point with.

When people discovered my half-finger hands, most of them turned away in embarrassment and either went quiet or started talking loudly about something completely different. I realized how difficult it was for most people to ignore physical disabilities, treat them like a natural thing, or simply to ask about them. I would have been glad to answer any question. Seeing someone grimace or stare out of curiosity without having the courage to ask me how I was—well, it hurt every time.

I was beginning to look at people differently, starting to grasp how many around me needed that extra bit of help, a little consideration and appreciation of the challenges they were facing. I used to see a blur on my way back from work, on the train, the bus, at the school gates, shopping, or driving down our street. Now I started seeing people. I saw the sad girl, the single mother, the lonely old man talking to himself. I saw the person with a different complexion who was frowned upon simply because of that, despite having been born in Denmark, or the political refugee trying to make sense of an affluent, but cold, country.

I noticed people moving away from the person in a wheelchair, those who stared at two women holding hands, shaking their heads at others for being who they were. I saw how many of us are different, how many of us faced everyday challenges. I saw how invisible these daily struggles could be to others. And I came to see how easy it was to make space for the differences, to reach out and to give myself in a smile, a nod, a silent demonstration that it was OK to be different, to take time, to be who we were.

My new exercise buddies made me appreciate another thing. I now belonged to a community. This came to me as quite a surprise. In my previous life I had never given it a thought that such communities existed, people who had nothing in common except they were brought together by accident, literally. Now I found myself sharing something with people who would otherwise have been completely invisible to me. We mostly came from different backgrounds; we had been doing completely different things in life before our paralysis; we lived in different parts of town, moved in different circles, had different friends.

But here we were. Twice a week, thrown together by a matter of chance, and what tied us together was the intensity of our experience and drive to recover; sharing something that only we could truly understand. While we could talk to our loved ones about what we had been through, they would never really understand what it had been, and was still, like. Our experiences were not something you could comprehend with your mind. You had to have been there, you had to have experienced it in your body. You had to have felt it, to have lived it and, in some cases, to have died.

In one way or another, we had all been there, on the other side of the tubes and wires, looking up from the bed. We had seen and felt the alarm and distress of our friends and relatives, breathed in the serious air of the doctors, the bustle of the nurses. We shared the existential fear in our bones, the sense that this is it, that life is or might soon be over.

We had stood on the edge of our lives, trying to come to terms with what might be. We had wrestled with wondering if it was OK to let go, to close our eyes and not know whether we would ever open them again. And then as we recovered, becoming well enough to know we had survived death, but somehow were still so weak our bodies failed to do the things they had always done.

And most of all, we all knew how it felt to live.

We were a mixed bunch. We would most likely never have met if it hadn't been for this. But now here we were, and I felt at home in their company. I laughed at the poor jokes we made about ourselves and everything we were unable to do. We were physically exhausted because of all the exercises, but also relaxed in each other's presence—at ease and comfortable. I could just be the person I had become with my crazy hair, bony body, and weak muscles.

The eight-year-olds in Daniel's classroom had asked all the obvious questions. The seventy-year-olds in the gym didn't have to. They already knew the answers.

On the days I wasn't with my new friends, I spent mornings and afternoons alone in the house. I saw our street, and the lives of my neighbors, from a different point of view. On either side of us lived widowers, both of their wives lost to painful cancer; one of them had had a bypass operation that had probably saved his life. They were both retired. I knew who they were, of course. I had talked to them and we had a perfectly friendly relationship; Peter had borrowed stuff from them for the garden. We were all good neighbors.

But I didn't know them, not really. Now we had something in common: time in the middle of the day and shared stories. It didn't take long for another pensioner a few houses down to come around, too. He had experienced a stroke. They came to see how I was, or if I needed any help, and before long I became part of their community. We all got along. They brought the coffee, and I set the table in the garden.

We talked about anything but being ill. We didn't have to. One could talk about how difficult it could be on certain days simply to get out of bed, to see the point of it all. And we all knew how that felt. But mostly we were just hanging out. They told me so many stories, from when they were young and had their lives ahead of them, all the recklessness and silliness of youth you tend to forget or never associate with elderly neighbors. Basically, we were having fun.

Peter and I had been so busy with our life, going to work, getting the children to school, sports, and after-school programs, that we hadn't really appreciated who our neighbors were. I now found myself a richer person through their company, their everyday generosity. I might have been on my own during the day, but like in the hospital, I realized I was never truly alone.

Life was different. There were so many things I had to think about, so many issues that needed to be solved. Peter drove me for check-ups at various hospitals, sometimes several times a week. We went to talk to a social worker from the city council who was assigned to my case, coordinating my continued physio and training. I was on extended sick leave from my job at the university, and I started to worry if I would ever be able to go back.

While I was still at the hospital, I had received a rather nice fellowship with excellent conditions for my research. They all knew what was going on with me and the fellowship was postponed accordingly. My new boss invited me for a chat. At first, I didn't want to go. I was nervous that I wouldn't be able to perform well and they might think me not worthy to return. This was all in my head. As it happens, my new boss was kindness itself, full of understanding for my situation and very generous. He wanted to say to me in person that he didn't expect to see me until I was ready—and then he wanted to give me an opportunity to see my new office.

That took me by surprise. It was a lovely day, warm and sunny, and as he opened the door and I walked into my office for the first time, I gasped. I could see the trees in the park right outside my window, the stream running through it. There was my desk and my chair. This was to be expected, of course, but they had also fitted in a couch for me to take a rest when I needed it. Everything was carefully planned for me to make a gradual transition back to work, one step at a time, at my own pace. I was so grateful, and I felt passionate about coming back to continue my scientific career. I was shown the way forward and I embraced it, happily.

It would take another six months before I was able to return to work, and then only part time. But I saw another target, and I aimed for it.

Slowly but surely, I was able to do more and more around the house. It wasn't easy not being able to do all the things I used to do, but I kept going even though I sometimes needed a break from everything. Peter and the children were all very helpful, but it didn't take away the pain and deep sorrow over what had happened to me and how it had affected the people I loved the most in this world.

One evening I decided to make dinner. I desperately wanted to get back to doing things I had always done, that I had never given a second thought to, and this felt like an easy way in. The rest of the family agreed to help getting me the ingredients I asked for. I didn't want to call on Peter for help, even though he was sitting in the study next door. I wanted to do this on my own. Tomatoes, garlic, onions, peppers, mushrooms, basil, lettuce and pasta: the simplest ingredients to put together. Or so I thought.

I joked to myself that I didn't have to be afraid of cutting off a fingertip. But it didn't help. It took me forever. The onions drove me crazy. I had no strength in my hands. I couldn't bend what was left of my fingers. I was getting exhausted from trying, frustrated from holding the knife with a tight, tiny grip; from rinsing the vegetables in excruciatingly cold water; from standing up. Some of my fingers started bleeding from the work. I was overwhelmed with how unfair it was. How difficult it was to resume living, and how it seemed it would always be.

I couldn't take it anymore, I couldn't help it. I stood there in front of the sink, feeling sorry for myself, locked in my own bubble of self-pity. Hating everything that had happened to me, hating every mountain I still had to climb to do all the things others never gave a thought to. I was tired of fighting. Tired of keeping going. Tired of everything.

I started crying. Standing there, overcome with grief, tears pouring down my cheeks. Miserable, disabled, and alone in my own world.

Then I felt his hand. Daniel just looked up at me, his tiny expressive face I knew so well.

"Mum," he said quietly. "I think you have the most beautiful hands in the world."

And after a very long and dark journey that started on New Year's Day, something deep inside of me finally came together. I was wrong. Life was not miserable. I might have lost a few pounds and limbs along the way, but in the way he looked at me, I realized I had gained so much more. I had added another layer to what it means to be human.

From that moment, I knew my life had changed for the better. Things were right.

That day, I healed.

Epilogue

I never thought I would write a book about myself, but five months in hospitals in 2013 profoundly changed my life and affected deeply how I think about myself and others. I will never be as strong as I used to be, and the active life I used to live is no longer an option. I have to take care of myself in a completely different way: I have to manage my schedule carefully and allow for breaks; I need my sleep and to be able to take an afternoon off at very short notice. If I am tired, I have to rest or my body will stop functioning.

I am practically blind in one eye and need glasses to read with the other. With a left thumb as my only unimpaired finger, I need to find alternative ways around most things. Simple tasks such as buttoning a shirt or tying my shoe laces take a lot longer now. Sometimes when things are getting too difficult, I look at my hands and curse everything that has happened to me.

Nothing prepared me for the speed of change in my life. It all came too fast and in the course of a single day, and it would probably have been so different if a doctor on night shift taking a home call hadn't mistaken a violent bacterial infection for the common flu and had got me to hospital much sooner. *Streptococcus pneumoniae* is one of the deadliest bacteria in the world: each year close to half a million children under five die from it worldwide, and yet many of us carry it without being harmed thanks to a healthy immune system.

It is spread by small droplets flying through the air from coughing and sneezing, and causes a range of illnesses such as ear and sinus infections and pneumonia, which can be serious enough, but what makes it particularly dangerous is its ability to penetrate barriers in the body, allowing it to enter into the blood or the tissue and fluids protecting the brain and the spinal cord, causing septicemia and meningitis. When this happens, the human body's natural protection is very limited. What separates a person from life or death at that critical stage can be down to a matter of minutes.

The bacteria shut me down. As with other patients who are locked in their own bodies, I was awake and conscious, but resembled a patient in a vegetative state. Studies have documented that it is often family members and not the medical staff who are the first to realize that patients are aware. This was certainly the case for me.

With the help of new communication technologies, we understand the long-term effects of being locked in better and have a new perspective on the quality of life a patient can experience, although no new technology has yet helped in the early stages, when most patients—like myself—are limited to blinking or eye movements. This is a most frustrating experience and the ultimate test of patience. Healthy people and medical professionals some-times assume that the quality of life of a patient who is locked in must be so poor that it is not worth continuing. But studies confirm that the majority of chronic patients profess to have a good quality of life, no worse than patients with severe disabilities, despite social isolation or difficulties with daily activities.

I know I was lucky. I got out and got my life back, even if it was a different life. Many don't. Every little sign, token, and recognition from people you love and care about mat-ters and increases your well-being as you lie there without speech or movement. You pay far more attention to the little things. They are all you have and they give you the strength to carry on.

That was how I felt. Being left alone for so many hours, locked in my body, the only thing I could do was think. In the beginning I couldn't even do that very well, as my

short-term memory was shot, but at least my shaky consciousness provided me with hope for starting life again.
We take for granted who we are, but without memories
we fade and if we lose control of the memories we have,
we lose all sense of who we are. Lying there, unable to
move, I had to figure out how to put myself back together
and as my mind became stronger, I found that I could
use my memories as building blocks; by placing them
carefully in the right order, one by one, I could remember
my own personal history and provide the all-important
key to my recovery.

Since my recovery, I have been asked over and over
what it feels like to be conscious and aware but unable to
communicate; to be paralyzed and understand what people were saying around me, but only able to move my eyes
from one side to the other—and blink. I hope I have given
you a sense of what it's like. If I were to sum it up in a single
word, it would be *loneliness*. I felt alone in the world, abandoned, let down, desperate and frightened. The worst part
was that I didn't know if I would remain like that, forever
entombed in my own body.

Having gone through this, I know that the final word I
would want to hear is a word of love. It is an often-used
cliché that in order to know what something is like, you
should try it yourself; and while I wouldn't want anyone
to experience what I have gone through, I do hope that

my story will inspire others to let those around you in need—from friends or family lying in a hospital bed, to colleagues or neighbors who have suffered in some way—know that they are not alone, that you care.

Every letter, postcard, flower, and token from family, friends and colleagues helped my recovery. They made me stronger and helped me fight the loneliness. There was no shortcut to getting my life back. I was forced to take the long road back to any sense of normality: two months in Intensive Care, three months at a rehabilitation center, followed by six months of training and recovery at a local rehabilitation center before I was able to work part time, and more than a year on top of that before I was back full time.

It was tough and it still is. I have learned that life can hurt in ways I wasn't even able to imagine. But I have also learned never to take anything for granted and that every day matters. In the face of death, I got a thirst for life, a strength to live and a sensitivity to enjoy even the simplest of everyday routines. In my hospital bed my constant refrain was "never mind," when Peter didn't get what I was trying to communicate. I've learned to be more patient with others and now if things don't go exactly as planned, or if someone does not entirely live up to what I'm expecting, I form the same words in my head: *Never mind.*

I am truly and deeply grateful for surviving, but I live with the consequences of what happened to me. My family suffered. We all have scars and we will have them forever. Not a day goes by without thinking about those consequences. Every day I'm reminded of the things I can't do anymore. And while I wish none of this had happened, life is curious. I have adapted to the change in my circumstances and learned to appreciate things that would not have happened had it not been for my illness.

I am still me, but I have changed. My priorities are different and some months after returning to continue my university career in data visualization, I realized that this was no longer what I wanted. It was a difficult decision. After all, I had worked very hard and for many years to get where I was. But now it felt natural to let go of it and do something else. In my job I talked mostly to my peers, my scientific colleagues, but now I wanted to make what I did with my life matter to more people. I had been given so much and now I wanted to pass it on.

As a scientist, I know that knowledge is the best weapon against disease and that ignorance is our greatest enemy. As a patient, I learned how critical it is in order to make a successful recovery to have some kind of control of your own situation and to be able to communicate properly. Knowledge and empowerment; I could work with that.

Just before I got ill I had been elected a Member of the Young Academy, at the Danish Royal Academy of Sciences and Letters. When I returned to work, I also returned to the Young Academy. Here I met like-minded spirits and together we founded an educational charity we call the Science Club, a mentoring network for children and young adults inspiring future scientists through scientific programs and creating role models within the natural sciences.

Our daughter Victoria had attended the Science Club for Girls in Boston. She loved it, but there was no similar program for her in Denmark, so I decided to start one up for her and as many other school children as possible.

Using my scientific skills to communicate complex data through easy graphics, I also founded a company, Graphicure, with a colleague from Boston. Our mission is to empower patients to monitor and understand their own treatment and recovery.

With the help of an incredible medical team who go to work every day to save lives, as well as the support of family, friends and colleagues, I didn't just get my life back. I got something more, something rare and of exceptional value: a profound desire to make my life matter, not only for me, but for as many as possible.

It was not simply my own life that had been affected by my illness. We sold our beloved house and moved into a flat. There was a lot of thinking about what we should do with our lives. Peter took a new job as a museum director and the children changed schools and made new friends.

We have always been close as a family, but now we are even closer. In the first few years following my recovery, they all stayed on high alert for every sign of me feeling unwell. I don't think that will ever go away. The shock sits with us as a family and it takes very little to take us back to where we were.

But this is also a strength, a compass for what we do, how we spend our time, and the choices we make. I can honestly say that it has increased our quality of life. What an utterly unexpected bonus. What we went through as a family was horrifying, terrible in all respects, but it has given us something positive we can use, and it made me realize that I can do something different with my life.

The Science Club was created to give future generations a better foundation for making a difference in the world. Graphicure was founded to allow patients to be people, to put control back into the hands of those who have lost it. And this book was written to give a voice to those who have none and for anyone whose life has changed out of all recognition from one moment to the next. I am trying to see my unexpected survival and recovery as a gift that can help others, too.

This is what I do. This is my life, and I am dedicating every moment to making it the best it can be.

A Caregiver's Checklist

All the months I spent in the hospital, and the time it took me to recover at home, taught me how lucky I was to have my family around me. They noticed all the little things and were in constant contact with nurses, therapists, and doctors—sharing what they had observed but also learning about my treatment. Their presence and advocacy made a difference and helped my way to recovery. If you have a loved one in the hospital in a critical condition or in a situation where she or he is not able fully to speak for her or himself, you must never lose sight of how important you are. You can make a difference.

There are many things you can do to help your loved one in these situations. I have collected a list—a caregiver's checklist—based on what Peter and the children did to make sure I made a better recovery, and on what gave them a sense of purpose when my future was uncertain.

1. *Be present and make your presence known.* This may sound self-evident. But it's not. As a relative you try not to be in the way of the doctors and nurses, you take a step back, you keep quiet, you don't want to disturb the treatment. Often, healthcare professionals too are trying in their own way to be as invisible as possible, to be nothing more than the anonymous treatment of a patient. But being invisible doesn't help anyone. The invisibility game makes communication terribly complicated. Therefore, what you need to do is to make yourself known. Make the healthcare staff know that you are there and ready to help in any way possible. You have something incredibly valuable to offer, the scarcest resource in any healthcare system: time.

2. *Learn to speak medical language and communicate your observations.* You're not a medical doctor, nurse, or therapist, and you're not supposed to be. But you need to learn and understand their language. You have to figure out how best to communicate with all healthcare staff. Use this knowledge to find the best way to share your own expertise, which will help foster a sense that you and the healthcare professionals are on the same team.

3. *Introduce the person. Make healthcare staff see beyond the patient.* No one knows the patient better than you.

You know their personal and/or work life before the illness, habits, likes and dislikes. You know their values and beliefs. Share that knowledge with the healthcare team in a way they will be able to understand. Bring photos and share stories that help them see the person lying there in the hospital bed.

4. *Record everything and keep track of changes.* Bring a notebook or a portable device to the bedside. Use it every day. Write everything down. Include things you don't think are necessary. Every incident and word. Every little detail. While sitting there by the bedside, you have all the time in the world. Use it to write down observations of all kind. What you see and hear. In particular, include the different things doctors and nurses say and do. There will be things you don't understand. Write it down for you to ask about or look into later. Write it down to note patterns, inconsistencies, and things you notice have a positive effect.

5. *Find allies.* You won't feel a special connection to every doctor or nurse caring for your loved one. Look toward healthcare professionals whom you immediately connect with, can relate to, and feel yourself bonding with. Talk to them. Draw them in and use them as a communication link to his or her colleagues. They will be a confidant with whom you can share more. With these allies, you and your observations will more likely be

incorporated into the treatment plan, and thus have a positive impact on the wellbeing of your loved one.

6. *Know that there are bad eggs.* I've met more doctors and nurses than the average patient and I am deeply and genuinely impressed with most of them. But I've also met a few who should not be in that profession. I've seen arrogance and ignorance at times when my health critically depended on the opposite. This is a very difficult topics to deal with, but you have to. If you see malpractice or negligence, call it out!

7. *Mistakes are made.* There is never enough time in any healthcare system. Doctors and nurses are busy and every single day they make multiple decisions under a lot of pressure. Sometimes they overlook things, not because they are not good at their jobs, but because of a stressful work environment. If you see things that doesn't seem right or pick up signals that staff don't seem to register, let them know. It may be nothing, but it could also be something that would profoundly change the health condition of your loved one.

8. *Be the eyes and ears of your loved one.* If you think you're struggling to comprehend what's going on with your loved one's health, imagine what he or she feels while lying in the hospital bed! Depending on the condition at hand the patient will be more or less cognizant of his or her situation, and you can play a key function as the

careful observant and memory of your loved one. While they are working hard to get well internally, help them retain a sense of the external world. Tell that person what's going on, explain details and do it with patience.

9. *If something goes wrong you are the memory and voice of your loved one.* All the things you have seen, written down, documented, felt, and talked about are useful if procedures fail. The better and more accurate your notes and observations are, the more meticulous you've been, and the more successful you've been in communicating with healthcare staff, the stronger your case will be if something goes seriously wrong and you have to deal with the legal system. You are, of course, trying anything in your powers to prevent that from happening, but sometimes even a single wrong call can have potentially fatal consequences. If a doctor on night duty on the day my illness broke out had sent me to the hospital immediately, I wouldn't have fallen ill, lost my fingers—or written this book. Luckily, Peter's detailed notes and recorded conversation with other healthcare professionals from that very same night helped to document the responsibility for the decisions that could have had a far worse outcome.

10. *Don't forget yourself.* You're important. Far more than you think. You need to take care of yourself or let others take care of you. People want to help. Accept what

they offer: a home-cooked meal, a talk on the phone or in person, or getting out of the hospital to go for a walk. Lean on the wider support network. It might be bigger than you think. When I gradually returned to conscious life I was surprised and overwhelmed by the many words and tokens of love and support, and so was Peter. This may just be what you need to go that extra mile that can save a life. I wouldn't be here if it weren't for others and for that I am forever grateful.

Acknowledgments

Surviving a full-scale pneumococcal infection with everything from the early stages of sinusitis and pneumonia to aggressive meningitis, sepsis, multi-organ failure and long-term coma is rare. Even more rare is it for a survivor to be able to tell her story. Following my recovery, I was met with a great professional interest from medical staff who wanted to know about all aspects of what it was like waking from a coma to being locked in, and how I responded to their care and treatment. I started a new research project and took on a PhD student to help specialists understand all aspects of how *Streptococcus pneumoniae* works.

In the process of all this, I realized that I was speaking on behalf of the many thousand voiceless patients who had experienced something similar, or related as long-term illness. I could use the combination of scientist and survivor to provide medical professionals with new knowledge and, equally important, to give significant others insight into what their loved ones go through. The doctors, nurses, and therapists who had treated me persuaded me that I had something to offer to science, to friends and relatives and to other patients like me.

Many asked me to tell my story, because, as they kindly put it, they thought it could help and inspire others who needed hope and support. This book is the result of that. The reception in the UK has been overwhelming. So many people have shared their own personal stories and told me how they have found courage and comfort in my story. I have been deeply moved by this. Responses from readers of all kinds have reaffirmed that writing this book was the right thing to do. It was only made possible by the encouragement and help of a lot of people to whom I am forever grateful.

I want to thank all the patients and staff I encountered along the way, named and unnamed in this book. I am deeply indebted to the doctors, nurses and therapists fighting next to me all the way to recovery with compassionate care, enormous strength, and professionalism. Besides the anonymous specialists in the ambulance, the talented staff at the local hospital, at the university hospital and at the rehabilitation center, four people in particular have played a critical part in my survival.

There are so many amazing doctors involved in any journey of recovery, too many to single out within my story, but I do especially want to mention my GP Thomas Clausen, who was the first person to save my life; had it not been for his experience and capacity, I would not have been here today. The second person to help save my life was chief physician Lisbeth Liboriussen at the ICU at the university hospital; she went beyond standard procedure to mend the woman in front of her. The third doctor to help save my life was the chief physician at Infectious Diseases at the university hospital, Merete Storgaard; she gave Peter and me a strong belief in being able to pull through, no matter what, and gave Peter a purpose by letting him into the science of my illness. The fourth person to help save my life was chief physician Anne Rasmussen at Hammel Neurorehabilitation and Research Center; she boosted my confidence and made me believe in my own recovery when she asked the simple question: "How do you do it?"

Apart from my family, only two people are named in the book. In respect of their privacy, both of their real names have been changed.

Thanks to my colleagues and friends all over the world from Palo Alto to Hong Kong, who helped me carry on and believe in the future: colleagues at Aarhus University, the national research center Pumpkin, the Department of Science Studies, the interdisciplinary nanoscience center iNANO and Aarhus Institute of Advanced Studies, where

I became a fellow while I was still in a coma; colleagues at *Dissertation Reviews,* some of whom I had never even met in person; colleagues at the MRC Mitochondrial Biology Unit in Cambridge and at Harvard Medical School in Boston. I would also like to extend my thanks to the Royal Danish Academy of Sciences and Letters, and the Young Academy.

I owe a special thanks to our neighbors, Eigil, Peter, and Poul, for their delightful company after my homecoming; to our friends, Graeme, Djuke, and Tony, who spent New Year's Eve with us just before all hell broke loose and followed my gradual recovery with the greatest concern; to Annemette for showing up in the time of need; and to Tine and Merete for their invaluable help and patience discussing medical facts.

Writing this book has been a long process for me from the very first draft chapters to the finished manuscript. A number of talented and inspiring people have encouraged me along the way. I am grateful to Donald Johanson as the first outside our little family to believe in the project and encourage me to get an agent; to Sterling Lord, who never stopped believing in the book and to my agent Antony Topping at Greene & Heaton for always looking out for me with impeccable judgement. Rowena Webb has been a wonderful editor, always giving me a confidence boost when I needed it. A special thanks to Gillian Stern for her valuable editorial work and enthusiastic support to the very end, and to the extraordinary team at Hodder & Stoughton for their great help. Also, thanks to everyone on my publishing team at The Experiment. Special thanks to Jennifer Kurdyla, my ever-patient editor, and Matthew Lore for advice and encouragement.

Bill Bryson has been the most wonderful mentor and friend one can imagine. Heartfelt thanks go out to my immediate family, my mother and sister, who took hundreds of hours out to visit me, my father, Peter's parents and sisters. I don't know where I would be without them. Thanks also to Peter's old friend, Thomas, who came down in the time of need as he always does, and my flock of aunts, who came to the rescue when none of us had the strength to do a belated spring cleaning of the house.

I have dedicated this book to my children, Daniel, Victoria, and Johan, who showed remarkable bravery and faith, and to Peter for being there—always. Peter gave me information when I had none. He was not only my emotional support, but also my main guide through this experience. Peter, in a sense, is how I came to understand what had happened, especially during the first crucial months when I was unaware of where I was, and was trying to regain memory and to understand how things had changed. It means everything to have support and love when you are fighting to get your life back.

About the Author

Rikke Schmidt Kjærgaard is a scientist, mother of three, and cofounder of Graphicure, a start-up company developing software solutions that empower patients to better understand their disease and manage treatment. She is also the cofounder and CEO of the Danish Science Club, a mentorship network for children and young adults. Prior to her illness, she was an associate professor at Aarhus University. She holds a PhD in science communication, with past positions as a postdoctoral fellow at MRC Mitochondrial Biology Unit in Cambridge, UK, and at Harvard Medical School. In 2012, she was elected Member of The Young Academy under the Royal Danish Academy of Sciences and Letters.